Everything You
Need to Know About
Enzymes

A Simple Guide to Using Enzymes to Treat
Everything from Digestive Problems and
Allergies to Migraines and Arthritis

Tom Bohager

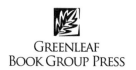

GREENLEAF
BOOK GROUP PRESS

Published by Greenleaf Book Group Press
4425 Mo Pac South, Suite 600
Longhorn Building, 3rd Floor
Austin, TX 78735

Distributed by Greenleaf Book Group LP

For ordering information or special discounts for bulk purchases, please contact Greenleaf Book Group LP at 4425 Mo Pac South, Suite 600, Longhorn Building, 3rd Floor, Austin, TX 78735, (512) 891-6100.

Design and composition by Greenleaf Book Group LP
Cover design by Greenleaf Book Group LP

Publisher's Cataloging-In-Publication Data
(Prepared by The Donohue Group, Inc.)

Bohager, Tom.
    Everything you need to know about enzymes : a simple guide to using enzymes
to treat everything from digestive problems and allergies to migraines and
arthritis / Tom Bohager. -- 1st ed.

        p. : ill. ; cm.

    Includes bibliographical references and index.
    ISBN: 978-1-929774-49-4

    1. Enzymes--Therapeutic use. 2. Dietary supplements. 3. Health. I. Title.
II. Title: Enzymes

RM666.E55 B645 2008
615/.35   2007941180

Printed in the United States of America on acid-free paper

08 09 10 11 12 13 14   10 9 8 7 6 5 4 3 2 1

First Edition

CONTENTS

• Bacterial Vaginosis • Bad Breath • Bedsores • Bladder Infection • Blood Cleanse • Bone Fractures • Bronchitis • Bursitis • Cancer • Candidiasis • Canker Sores • Celiac Disease • Cholesterol (Elevated) • Chronic Fatigue Syndrome • Circulation (Poor) • Colds • Colic (Infantile) • Colitis, Ulcerative • Constipation • Cramps (Muscle) • Crohn's Disease • Cystic Fibrosis • Dandruff • Decubitus Ulcers • Depression • Dermatitis • Diabetes • Diarrhea • Diverticulosis/Diverticulitis • Dyspepsia • Ear Infection • Eczema • Edema (Water Retention) • Endocrine Glands (Support) • Energy/Endurance • Environmental Toxicity • Epstein-Barr Virus • Erectile Dysfunction • Exercise • Eye Conditions • Fatigue • Fever • Fibromyalgia • Flatulence • Flu • Fungus • Gallbladder Imbalances • Gastritis • Gastroesophageal Reflux Disease • Gingivitis • Gluten Intolerance • Gout • Gum Problems • Hair Loss • Halitosis • Hangover • Hay Fever • Headache • Heartburn • Hemorrhoids • Herpes Virus • Herpes Zoster (Shingles) • Hiatal Hernia • High Blood Pressure • Hot Flashes • Hormonal Imbalances • Hypertension • Hypoglycemia • Hypothyroidism • Indigestion • Infection • Inflammatory Bowel Disease • Influenza • Insect Bites and Stings • Insomnia • Irritable Bowel Syndrome • Joint Pain • Jock Itch • Kidney Stress • Lactose Intolerance • Laryngitis • Liver Toxicity • Longevity • Lupus • Lyme Disease • Lymphatic Congestion • Malabsorption Syndrome • Menopause • Migraines • Mucus Congestion • Multiple Sclerosis • Nausea • Nervousness • Osteoporosis • Oxidative Stress • Parasites • Peptic Ulcer • Periodontal Disease • Pituitary Imbalances • Premenstrual Syndrome • Prostate Disorders • Psoriasis • Respiratory Ailments • Rheumatism • Ringworm • Shingles • Sinusitis • Skin Problems • Skin Ulcers • Sleep • Sports Injury • Strains • Stress • Sugar Intolerances • Surgery • Systematic Lupus Erythematosus • Thyroid Imbalance • Tinnitus • Triglycerides (Elevated) • Ulcers • Vaginitis • Viral Infections • Water Retention • Weight Control • Yeast Infection

INTRODUCTION

Surely you know someone who seems to have boundless energy, rarely gets sick, and apparently escapes the damage of passing time. We say these people are the fortunate ones, blessed with good genes, genes that keep them healthy, strong, fit, looking young, and happy. But only a small part of their good fortune can be genetic. (Some researchers believe that genetics only account for 5 to 15 percent of the factors that determine lifespan.) In actuality, our health and the length of our life are primarily determined by the availability of metabolic energy. Though this availability is partially attributed to what we inherit genetically, the factors include how we live, where we live, what we eat, how much we eat, how much we exercise, and what we do for work, to name a few. In other words, our life choices, our circumstances, and our environment determine, to the greatest degree, the quality of our health and length of our life.

Regardless of the choices you are making now, though, there is little doubt that you want to be healthy and live a long life without greatly inconveniencing yourself or your loved ones. Well, you can!

A NEW PATH

Often we think of life as a journey. Where we end up depends on the path we have chosen. Every week you make hundreds of choices about your journey, and your choices affect your health. But the path you are currently on is probably convenient for you and brings you some measure of pleasure. The food, alcohol, snacks, TV, where you live . . . the list goes on. Think of what you are about to learn as a parallel path: not one that takes you in a completely different direction, but rather a slight alteration to the path you have already chosen. Yes, it's new in some ways, but not unfamiliar; the direction is the same but the journey lasts longer and is more enjoyable. The change I'm recommending is defined by a newfound knowledge of what is ultimately burning up your health and potential years, exhausting your metabolic energy—enzyme deficiencies and imbalances.

The new direction makes use of a simple, natural method for improving your health dramatically without going to extremes in altering your lifestyle. It can revitalize your body, renew your energy, and ease your health complaints, but it's not a miracle drug. In this book, I will reveal how simple the path to good health can be—all because of the power of enzymes, the amazing proteins that support the basic metabolic and digestive processes that make life possible.

Enzymes are the providers of metabolic energy (or cellular energy); they play a vital role in digestion, our immune system, our vitality, the aging process, and literally every function of the body. Our bodies produce trillions of enzymes to support these functions, but the vast majority of us find ways to derail that production process through poor life choices. As a result we make fewer enzymes than our body requires, and suddenly our body is struggling to support some of the primary functions necessary to sustain life. We feel tired and lethargic, the toll of aging becomes more pronounced, and we get sick.

Research has shown that by supporting the body's mechanisms for producing enzymes and by taking enzyme supplements, we can reduce the negative effects of stressors on our bodies. These supplements are readily available, comparatively inexpensive, and all natural. Yet they will improve health, longevity, and well-being in ways that are superior to supplemental vitamins, minerals, and herbs.

HOW THIS BOOK CAN HELP

This book will help you appreciate the importance of enzymes and how vital they are in supporting optimal health. Once you truly understand this connection, you will have a potent tool to help you maintain your health and overcome common health issues.

In part 1, I will explain the vital contribution enzymes make to our overall health, vitality, and longevity. Chapter 1 describes the role of enzymes as the catalysts of life, explaining how they are produced and used by the body. Chapter 2 explains the link between enzymes and digestive health. Chapter 3 identifies how enzymes help to defend against and overcome poor health and disease. Chapter 4 offers simple solutions for incorporating enzymes into your daily life for a fast and effective path to better health—no matter what your health issues.

In part 2, I offer enzyme therapy recommendations for treating specific illnesses and ailments, covering everything from acne and athlete's foot to thyroid imbalance and viral infections.

Enzymes have changed the lives of millions of people, and they can change yours too. Whether you're in good health now, you have a few health complaints, or you've been living with pain or discomfort for a long time, the information and programs recommended in this book can help you improve your quality of life and feel better than you may have ever believed possible.

PART ONE:
ENZYME ESSENTIALS

CHAPTER ONE

HOW ENZYMES AFFECT OUR HEALTH

Imagine giving up forty years of life. For some unexplained reason we just decide that we don't need the extra time. Though this seems absurd, it is in effect what many of us do. What a shame it would be if we had the potential to live to be 110 but instead only lived to be 70. What if instead of losing years of life we lost precious quality of life? Perhaps we could live healthily, happily, and with little evidence of aging, but instead we felt tired, old, or sick. The fact is that we all have a life potential that extends well beyond the years we will actually live and the quality of life we actually enjoy.

In order for us to live to our full potential, we would have to make all of the right choices from birth (or our parents would have to make all of the right choices for us). We would probably have to sacrifice where we want to live, what we want to eat, and what we do for work and play to achieve our maximum life potential. Of course, not only do we choose not to follow that path, it would be impossible even if we tried. But that doesn't mean we can't improve, enrich, and extend our health and our energy now without making drastic changes in lifestyle.

Life potential varies in each of us, but it is directly related to the amount of metabolic energy that we have at our disposal (Roy Walford, *Beyond the 120 Year Diet*, New York: Four Walls Eight Windows, 2000, 63–66). There is only so much energy our cells can express in our lifetime, and when that energy is gone, so are we. We can burn up this energy fast or make it last—the choice is ours!

The key to maximizing metabolic energy, or what some call metabolic efficiency, which directly affects our life and health, is enzymes—the unique proteins that break down our food and convert it into energy. Enzymes have been called the "catalysts of life" and have many uses, some occurring in the body naturally, some contained in the raw foods we eat, and others as supplements to make up for what the body lacks. Used properly, they can increase the metabolic energy available to our bodies, decrease our susceptibility to disease, ease scores of common ailments, and increase our life potential. If you want to understand how, read on.

WHAT ARE ENZYMES?

Enzymes are defined as protein catalysts since they are made up of amino acids, just as proteins are. However, enzymes are unique, because they are biologically active—they contain energy. It is this energy that makes it possible for enzymes to perform the work of life. The energy contained in enzymes is not unlimited, however. Rather, an enzyme works until all of its energy is exhausted—you might say it wears out. Once the enzyme no longer contains any biological activity, it ceases being a catalyst and becomes like any other protein, ready to be absorbed by the body.

There are two types of enzymes our bodies naturally produce: Digestive enzymes are responsible for the digestion of food, the assimilation of its nutrients into our bodies, and the elimination of its nonessential and toxic ingredients. Metabolic enzymes are the ones that make every biochemical reaction possible within each of our 100 trillion cells. These biochemical reactions provide the metabolic energy that ultimately allows us to see, hear, breathe, feel, walk, and talk. Simply put, without enzymes, life would not exist!

DIGESTIVE ENZYMES

Think about your last meal. The food you ate contained vitamins, minerals, proteins, fats, and sugars. Our bodies convert the nutrients in the food we eat into energy, but the nutrients must be unlocked from their sources before our bodies can benefit from them. Without enzymes, these reactions would occur far too slowly for the body to sustain life. By definition enzymes instigate or enhance biochemical reactions—catalysts—and they speed up this process dramatically.

Consider your typical nutritional bar (or if you prefer, candy bar). Nutrients in the bar can provide energy to the body, but they must be unlocked before we can utilize them. A random chemical process could take years to break down the nutrients in the bar and release the energy. A catalyst (digestive enzyme) will speed up this process dramatically by reducing the amount of time it takes to start the process of releasing energy. Instead of years, it takes hours.

Supplemental enzymes (the kind you would find in a health food store) are able to support the digestive process in the same way as those naturally produced in our bodies. When digestive enzyme supplements are consumed with food, the need for the body to produce digestive enzymes decreases, preventing our bodies from having to use up nutrients and energy to provide them. This simple solution increases the benefit we get from food and the efficiency of our digestive systems. As you will soon see, this in turn will benefit our health in major ways, adding to our quality of life and well-being.

METABOLIC ENZYMES

Enzymes that are active and functional in the cells, tissues, or bloodstream are called metabolic enzymes. Though you might have heard about the importance of digestive enzymes, very few people know about or can accurately describe the role of metabolic enzymes. Metabolic enzymes are any enzymes produced within the body that are not used for digestion. They are the enzymes that make biochemical reactions for detoxification and energy production (metabolic energy) possible within the cells. They have been called the spark of life, the energy of life, and the vitality of life.

Every organ, every bit of tissue, and all of the 100 trillion cells in our body depend upon the reaction of metabolic enzymes and their energy factor. You may wonder why it is that few of us have ever heard of metabolic enzymes, since they have such an important role within the body. The reason is that these enzymes cannot be produced in a lab, encapsulated, bottled, and sold to you, the consumer. They can only be produced by the cells within the body.

In his book *For the Love of Enzymes: The Odyssey of a Biochemist*, Arthur Kornberg, winner of a Nobel Prize in medicine for his study of enzymes, writes, "By 1982 some 1,400 diseases, each due to a defect in a single gene, had been described in medical literature . . . For most of the diseases, the biochemical basis is still unknown. For approximately 200 of them, the disease is known to be due to a deficiency or malnutrition of a single enzyme." Since 1982 many more diseases have been attributed to such a deficiency.

If we could somehow identify the metabolic enzyme needed for a specific health issue, manufacture it, and deliver it to the cell, metabolic enzyme pills would be in every health food store and pharmacy in the world and would no doubt be contributing to the prevention and reversal of many of the most fatal diseases known to man. But even without that technology, we can use enzyme supplements to support the body's ability to produce metabolic enzymes—it's a key focus of this book.

A third type of enzymes, food enzymes, are active in raw food. Though these are not produced by the body, they are beneficial to the digestive process. I speak more about them in chapter 2.

ENZYME POTENTIAL

Dr. Edward Howell, in his book *Enzyme Nutrition*, explains that we are all born with a different potential for producing enzymes. Enzyme potential is the number of enzymes we have the ability to produce in our lifetime, whether metabolic or digestive. The more digestive enzymes your body is forced to manufacture to digest the food you consume, the fewer metabolic enzymes it will have the ability to produce. This leads to an enzyme shortage and the quickest path to disease and a shortened life span. Dr. Howell illustrates this by suggesting we have a kind of enzyme bank account from which we make constant withdrawals; the fewer withdrawals, the longer we live. Some have described this process by saying that the body will borrow metabolic enzymes to manufacture digestive enzymes and vice versa.

Dr. Howell's theory has caused some debate, however. Because of the specific functions enzymes perform, it's impossible for the body to borrow metabolic enzymes to use in the digestive process. However, from puberty on, with each passing decade, our bodies produce approximately 10 to 13 percent fewer enzymes than the previous decade. Dr. Howell references numerous studies in humans, insects, and animals that all show a decrease in enzyme output with age.

Regardless of the debate over Dr. Howell's explanation of enzyme potential, if we consider that our bodies require energy and there is only so much energy to go around, it seems fairly clear that the more energy you expend digestively, the less energy you will have metabolically. Roy Walford, MD, described this as operating at maximum metabolic efficiency. He was able to dramatically increase the lifespan of mice in his lab at UCLA by reducing the daily requirement of digestive energy. He did this by restricting the calorie intake of the mice (see appendix D). This is why I prefer the terms *"energy potential"* or *"life potential"* to *"enzyme potential."*

PRIMARY ENZYME CATEGORIES

Researchers have been able to identify and name more than five thousand enzymes that our bodies manufacture and use, but there are likely far more, perhaps tens of thousands of different enzymes within the body. Why are there so many? Our bodies depend on so many enzymes because each enzyme has a particular and limited function, a specific job, and it can do nothing else. A protein is made up of many amino acids, sometimes thousands, all bound together in a long chain. A particular enzyme can alter that protein by breaking certain links or bonds in the chain, but that enzyme can only break the chain in those very specific locations. A different enzyme is required to continue the job, breaking different links in the chain. Then a third, fourth, fifth, sixth enzyme takes over, until the protein no longer exists. In its place

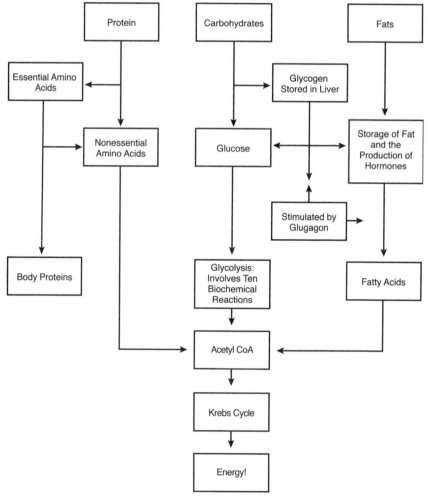

How carbohydrates, fats, and proteins are used by our bodies

we have thousands of amino acids, unattached and unbound, ready for use by the body as the building blocks of tissue.

Because there are so many individual enzymes, they are categorized by the type of chemical reaction they catalyze. Although there are many different categories, the most important categories in terms of digestion and enzyme therapy are proteases, lipases, and carbohydrases. Each of these categories plays a specific role metabolically and digestively. Proteases break down (hydrolyze) proteins, lipases break down lipids (fats), and carbohydrases break down carbohydrates. Within each of these categories there are perhaps thousands of enzymes. A fourth type of enzyme that plays an important role in our bodies is cellulase, the enzyme that breaks down cellulose (fiber). Though cellulase is technically a carbohydrase (cellulose is a carbohydrate), it is the only enzyme our body does not have the ability to manufacture. Occasionally this enzyme is put into a separate category.

Proteases break down proteins.

Lipases break down lipids, or fats.

Carbohydrases break down carbohydrates.

Cellulases (technically a form of carbohydrase) break down cellulose.

Think of enzymes as tools, with each tool having a slightly different function. You would never use a screwdriver to drive a nail into a piece of lumber. It's the same with the different categories of enzymes. Carbohydrases can never break down proteins; their specific function is to break down carbohydrates. However, sometimes the relationship between tools is much closer. Wrenches can look alike, but they come in different sizes. No matter how hard you try, a half-inch wrench will not fit a one-inch bolt. So, even though there are similarities between the enzymes within the categories, they each have a slightly different purpose: each fits a different size bolt, figuratively speaking. We need many different kinds of enzymes to break down the many different substances in our food and to speed up the many different biochemical reactions in each of our cells.

ENZYMES AND ILLNESS

Here is the simplest of truths regarding your health and enzymes: If you want to stay healthy, you need to support the body's mechanism for producing digestive and metabolic enzymes. All disease is the result of a deficiency or imbalance of some kind, a lack of something essential to health that results in sickness and pain. By bringing the body back into balance, you can improve your health and avoid disease. Enzymes are what help the body achieve such balance.

I have already mentioned Arthur Kornberg, who won a Nobel Prize in medicine for his study of enzymes. In 1982 he identified more than two hundred diseases directly attributed to a "deficiency or malnutrition of a single enzyme." For instance, a deficiency in the enzyme G6PD (glucose-6-Phosphate Dehydrogenase)—the most common human enzyme deficiency, with some 400 million people worldwide affected (Scriver et al., 1995)—is associated with neonatal jaundice and hemolytic anemia. Some G6PD deficient individuals are also allergic to fava beans (Carson et al., 1956; Beutler, 1994).

To better illustrate the important role enzymes play in supporting health, let's take a look at the enzyme protease, which is one of the most important types of enzymes in terms of a healthy immune system. The immune system is the body's defense system (see appendix C for additional information). The immune system's ability to fight off invaders depends on the enzyme protease, which breaks down proteins. Most types of illness are in some way related to protein. For example, cancer cells are surrounded by the protein fibrin. The blood clots that cause stroke and a high percentage of heart attacks are made up of this same protein. Pathogenic bacteria and parasites are comprised of proteins. Viruses are enveloped by protein, and fungal forms such as *Candida* contain a protein nucleus surrounded by a chitin shell (see CANDIDIASIS in part 2). Therefore, we need a plentiful supply of protease to overcome protein invaders in the body that will make us ill if left unchecked.

If you seem to catch every virus that comes your way, it's very possible that your immune system is underactive because of a deficiency in metabolic protease, a key component of the white blood cells that attack and destroy viruses. We are equipped to have a strong, healthy system. "Our immune system is overbuilt for success," according to Ellen Cutler, MD, author of *Micro Miracles: Discover the Healing Power of Enzymes.* Unfortunately, we can inhibit our immune system's abilities by placing too high a demand elsewhere.

Some very convincing research shows that the greater the burden we place on the digestive system, the less effective and active our immune system becomes. When we eat, digestion becomes the priority. Our body will always supply the energy our digestive system needs to benefit from the food we have eaten, no matter how little that leaves for other systems. Perhaps you have experienced this when, after a large meal, it takes all the energy you can muster just to stay awake. That energy demand robs all other systems of the body of the vital energy they need to keep up.

Thus it should not surprise us to learn that when we eat cooked and processed foods, especially when we overeat, our immune system actually becomes less active. The protease production so essential to immune support decreases since the energy required to manufacture these enzymes has been dedicated to producing digestive enzymes. We pay the price initially by being tired, but over time by suffering from poor health. If the pattern persists over years, our body may no longer be able to keep up on a regular basis; a shortage of certain metabolic enzymes (metabolic energy) will then occur, and eventually take its toll. However, we do not call it an enzyme deficiency—we have given it other names, like diabetes, cancer, heart disease, and lupus.

The environment within our body also affects the functionality of the enzymes we produce and consume. Enzymes function properly within specific environments and variations from their optimal surroundings, particularly in pH (acidity or alkalinity) and temperature, can decrease or increase their ability to catalyze biochemical reactions. Enzymes can become less active, inactive, or denatured in suboptimal settings. When inactive, an enzyme is not acting on, catalyzing, or digesting anything. When it is returned to its proper environment, it will likely become active again. When denatured, an enzyme loses all activity and can no longer serve as a catalyst under any condition. If our bodies are not in balance (for instance, the pH in our small intestines is too acidic) the enzymes we produce or consume may do us little good. The importance of pH will be discussed in more detail in chapter 3.

USING SUPPLEMENTAL ENZYMES TO IMPROVE HEALTH

As discussed, metabolic enzyme production (or the lack of it) plays a surprisingly important role in maintaining good health. Unfortunately, when metabolic enzyme production suffers there is no pill that can specifically make up for the loss or lack of these vital metabolic enzymes directly. However, though we may not be able to replace the enzymes we are specifically deficient in with supplements, we can supply the body with the energy and resources it needs to rectify the deficiency and achieve the balance that is lacking.

The importance of metabolic energy is perhaps better understood through the research of J.W. MacArthur and W.H.T. Baillie, who studied the life span of the Daphinia water flea. They concluded that the duration of the insect's life varied with the intensity of its metabolic needs. (Edward Howell, *Enzyme Nutrition* [New York: Avery, 1995] 22). At lower temperatures the metabolic enzymes worked at a slower rate and the insect lived five times longer (108 days at 46 degrees) than in higher temperature environments (25 days at 82 degrees). As enzymes did their work, the insect's enzymatic potential was depleted. From their research MacArthur and Baillie concluded that we are all born with a fixed capacity to make metabolic enzymes.

Though this example is a bit simplistic, it gives us a glimpse of one of life's truths: metabolic energy, made possible by metabolic enzymes, dictates life span. By decreasing the demand on our bodies to use metabolic energy for digestion, we have the ability to ration our energy to extend life and health.

Therefore, one of the most effective ways to improve your health is to use supplemental digestive and therapeutic enzymes. (Please note that the recommendations in this book are in no way intended to replace recommendations or advice from physicians or other health care providers. They are intended to support your path to optimal health. If you suspect you have a medical problem, I urge you to seek medical attention from a competent health care provider.) The main difference between supplemental digestive enzymes and supplemental therapeutic enzymes (or what some people call systemic enzymes) is not necessarily the enzymes themselves, but timing. Taken at different times, in different situations, each enzyme can have different effects. When taken at the beginning of a meal, the enzymes will assist the digestive process by breaking down the food. When taken apart from meals on an empty stomach, they can be absorbed by the body to be utilized systemically or therapeutically. In enzyme therapy, though, it is crucial to begin with the digestive process. Though the digestive process requires an incredible amount of energy under normal circumstances, the demand increases when poor food choices are made due to the type or quantity of food consumed. Improving digestion by taking a digestive enzyme supplement ensures that your body will benefit from the nutrients in the food you consume and it has the energy it needs to maintain the other systems, particularly when you're ill and the other systems aren't functioning as efficiently as they could be.

Then the next step is to determine which category of enzymes will assist you therapeutically in overcoming the most obvious deficiency to produce the fastest results. Therapeutic enzymes are much less effective if an individual is not taking digestive enzymes or in some other way resting the digestive system by fasting, improving food choices, or reducing calories. The reason for this is that the enzymes intended to provide a therapeutic effect by being absorbed into the blood actually begin digesting the food in the gut and as a result become less potent. This is especially true if a person is in the middle of a health crisis. For therapeutic enzymes to have a healing effect, it is imperative that there is not a heavy demand for digestive energy.

When enzymes are taken to achieve a therapeutic effect, they are taken on an empty stomach (a half hour before or two hours after consuming food). They are not intended to help digest food. Instead they are absorbed into the blood and can benefit different systems of the body, such as the cardiovascular system by increasing circulation, the immune system by providing it with essential enzymes to manufacture healthy white blood cells, and the endocrine system by taking stress off of the glands.

Though enzyme supplements may not function directly as metabolic enzymes, they have been shown to improve metabolic function. The therapeutic or systemic use of enzymes is designed specifically to *support* a deficiency in metabolic enzymes, not replace them. Each enzyme category can address specific deficiencies; if the deficiency is corrected, many health issues can be corrected as well.

The question then becomes, how do supplemental enzymes help with a metabolic enzyme deficiency since individual enzymes have such specific applications?

Let's look at the immune system again for two possible explanations. The first is that the supplemental enzymes (proteases in this case) act as raw material from which the lymph system and bone marrow can manufacture additional white blood cells. The second is that the protease begins digesting dead and damaged cells—which are primarily made up of protein—throughout the body, reducing the need for metabolic protease elsewhere. By lessening the demand, the supplemental proteases allow proteases that would have been produced for these purposes to be employed as part of the immune system.

This is just one example of how enzymes can be used therapeutically. Now let's look deeper into the therapeutic uses of specific types of enzymes.

PROTEASES

As mentioned above, proteases play a key role in supporting immune function, but this category of enzymes does so much more. This is why it is the most widely researched type of enzyme in the world. Proteases, or proteolytic enzymes as they are sometimes called, are those that break down proteins. When proteolytic enzymes are consumed with food, they assist in breaking down the proteins we have eaten, such as steak, fish, and eggs. When taken between meals, their role changes significantly; they assist with immune imbalances, heavy metal toxicity, inflammatory conditions, circulatory disorders, skin problems, constipation, water retention, inappropriate blood clots, heart disease, stroke, and cancer, among other health problems. The use of proteases for these conditions is the second most popular use of enzyme therapy after digestive applications. The logical reasons for their popularity are their many applications and the direct connection between proteins and illness.

There are several different types of protease used therapeutically, derived from four main forms:

- Fungal-based, sometimes called plant-based: protease, catalase, and seaprose
- Bacterial-based: serratiopeptidase and nattokinase
- Plant-sourced (sometimes called "tropical"): bromelain, papain, and ficin
- Animal-sourced: pancreatin, trypsin, and chymotrypsin

Most of these will be discussed in more detail in chapter 4.

FUNGAL- OR PLANT-BASED LIPASES

The second most researched group of enzymes is lipases. These enzymes are lipolytic, which means that they break down or disengage fat. Lipases are found in both plant-based and animal-sourced enzymes. They are one of the simplest enzymes to understand and one of the easiest to recommend, as they are effective for many issues related to fats. For example, many researchers believe that obesity can be traced to a lipase deficiency. One study showed that 100 percent of clinically obese individuals (whose weight is 30 percent greater than their ideal body weight) are lipase deficient (H. Santillo, *Food Enzymes: The Missing Link to Radiant Health* [Prescott, AZ: Hohm Press 1993], 36).

Fat is found in our cells, skin, blood (as HDL and LDL cholesterol), and the sheath that surrounds our nerves. Fat also plays a crucial role in hormone production. Additionally, the fat-soluble vitamins A, D, E, and K require lipase in order to be absorbed in the body. For all of the above reasons, lipase is recommended therapeutically for high cholesterol, obesity, high triglycerides, heart disease, hormonal imbalances, nerve problems, fat-soluble vitamin deficiencies, and skin problems such as eczema and psoriasis.

CARBOHYDRASES

Carbohydrases break down carbohydrates. This category is a bit more complicated because carbohydrates are a broad category that includes sugars, fiber, complex carbohydrates, and cellulose.

Basic carbohydrases, often called amylases, help to break down complex carbohydrates such as those in fruits, vegetables, and legumes into simple sugars. Therapeutically, these amylases have been shown to regulate histamine, which is produced by cells in the body when a perceived invader is recognized. Histamine is responsible for the common allergy symptoms many people experience when the pollen count in the air is high. Though it is difficult to say exactly how amylase is involved in this process, it is believed to simply break histamine down. So when the body produces histamine in defense of an intruder it incorrectly perceives as harmful, the enzyme amylase is there to curb its effect. Others have suggested that amylase helps the body identify allergens as nonharmful, and thus actually avoid producing the histamine. I suspect it is a bit of both. (See L. Desser, A. Rehberger, "Induction of tumor necrosis factor in human peripheral-blood mononuclear cells by proteolytic enzymes," *Oncology* 47 (1990): 475–77.)

Carbohydrases are also good at raising blood sugar. The carbohydrases from fungal sources are amylase, maltase, glucoamylase, alpha-galactosidase, hemicellulase, xylanase, pectinase, and phytase. If you have sugar cravings, food cravings, and low blood sugar, amylase in particular may help tremendously.

The carbohydrase enzymes that digest sugars are involved in breaking down sucrose, lactose, and maltose. When these sugars are not properly digested, people often exhibit symptoms of depression, panic attacks, severe mood swings or mania, abdominal cramps, diarrhea, and environmental sensitivities. The sugar-digesting carbohydrases from fungal (plant-based) sources are sucrase, lactase, and maltase.

The carbohydrases that digest fiber are called cellulases, and they are the only digestive enzymes our body does not manufacture, although the friendly bacteria in our intestinal tract do produce cellulase for our benefit (see chapter 3).

PLANT-BASED VS. ANIMAL-SOURCED ENZYMES

You may have noticed a few references so far to the source of particular enzymes. Enzymes primarily come from four sources: fungus, bacteria (mainly probiotics), animals, or plants. There are really two schools of thought when it comes to enzyme therapy, and they differ primarily on the source of the enzymes. The first school hypothesizes that enzymes derived from animals are superior in overcoming a health crisis. The second school proclaims that plant-based enzymes (fungal and bacterial) have the advantage.

ANIMAL-SOURCED ENZYME THERAPY

Animal-sourced enzymes have been studied since the late nineteenth century (see appendix D). There is great interest in this form of therapy, and particularly in the proteases pancreatin, trypsin, and chymotrypsin. Research has focused heavily on how these enzymes affect cancerous tumors. Cancer cells are surrounded by a protein that protects them by disguising them from the immune system. These enzymes break down that protein and expose the cancer to the immune system for removal. These enzymes may have a similar effect on viruses and bacteria.

The other areas of research on the health benefits of these enzymes include inflammation, heart disease, and stroke. The protein fibrin contributes to these conditions by causing blood clots. By removing excess fibrin, these proteases reduce inflammation and the risk of inappropriate blood clots, which greatly limits the risk of heart disease or stroke. By some estimates more than $50 million has been spent researching the benefits of these animal-sourced enzyme products. The evidence of their efficacy, in the form of studies, patents, pharmaceutical drugs, and credible research, is indisputable.

Though there are obvious benefits to the animal-sourced enzyme approach, there are also some potential problems. First, people who are vegan or vegetarian will not want to take this form of supplement, since it originates with animals that must be slaughtered to extract the raw material. Second, slaughterhouse animals often come from questionable sources and have questionable health and diets, and the use of steroids, antibiotics, and the like is prevalent in raising farm animals today. Thus, many choose to stay away from enzyme supplements from this source.

Third, enzyme potency is determined by how much protein, fat, or carbohydrates the enzyme can break down, and animal-sourced enzymes are relatively weak when compared to plant-sourced and -based enzymes. In fact, when animal proteases were tested against plant-based proteases under the same conditions, the plant-based enzymes broke down between ten and one hundred times more protein per milligram than the animal-sourced enzymes, depending on the protein. (It should be noted that this test was limited and it is possible the animal-based enzymes may outperform plant-based enzymes when exposed to different proteins.)

It stands to reason that the higher the proteolytic activity, the more effective the product. For this reason, the number of tablets that some people using animal-sourced enzyme supplements have to consume per day to achieve the therapeutic effects ranges from thirty to ninety. For most people this does not seem practical, especially since they are most likely taking other supplements and medications as well.

One must acknowledge that there are probably unknown factors associated with the success of the research on animal-sourced proteolytic enzymes. It's possible that their effectiveness is based on more than just the proteolytic activity. For example, in individuals who have extreme organ or gland deficiencies (pancreatitis, pancreatic cancer, liver cancer, gall bladder failure, or the like), animal-sourced enzymes seem to fortify the glands and organs in ways that the plant-based enzymes cannot. It is what we call the "law of similar," which is the basis of homeopathy. This theory states that even though the source is animal and not human, the body recognizes it as similar. Because of this, when animal-sourced enzymes are ingested, the body is able to recognize from which gland or organ the animal-sourced enzyme originated; thus the body is able to use this source to fortify glands and organs more effectively. Because of this connection, it is often recommended that individuals diagnosed with cancer of an organ or gland deficiency (who are not vegetarian or vegan) take both plant-based and animal-based enzymes.

PLANT-BASED ENZYME THERAPY

Plant-based enzymes taken from fungi and bacteria currently represent about 80 percent of all of the enzymes sold in health food stores. The remaining 20 percent is made up of a combination of animal-sourced enzymes, such as pancreatin and trypsin, and plant-sourced enzymes such as bromelain and papain. Plant-based enzymes most often originate from a fungus called aspergillus. This fungus produces a large amount of enzymes, including proteases, lipases, amylases, and cellulases, naturally active in a broad pH range. The enzymes are often called fungal or microbial enzymes. However, most people in the nutrition industry refer to them as plant-based, since the aspergillus is grown in a lab on different plants that serve as its food source. One of the benefits of using aspergillus is that it can be manipulated to manufacture different types of enzymes by changing the type of aspergillus used, the plant's food source, or the temperature, humidity, pH, or environment.

There are a number of benefits inherent in plant-based enzyme therapy:

- The enzymes are vegetarian and vegan and can thus be consumed by everyone.

- They are generally the most potent source of enzymes, between ten and one hundred times more effective at digesting proteins, fats, and carbohydrates per milligram than animal enzymes.

- Unlike animal sources, the health of the source is never questionable.

- The pH range is broad, making them active in stomach acid and throughout the rest of the body.

For all of the above reasons, plant-based enzymes are often the first choice in addressing health issues and/or enzyme deficiencies.

Now that you have the foundational knowledge of enzymes that you need to understand how they are tied to our health and longevity, we can explore how enzymes are used in specific treatments.

CHAPTER TWO
ENZYMES AND DIGESTION

Since digestion is the most energy-consuming function our body performs, it stands to reason that altering food intake or altering the demand placed on the digestive system will result in significant changes (good or bad) to overall health. Between 60 to 80 percent of the body's energy is used to move food through the digestive system, maintain balance between the acidity of the stomach and the alkalinity of the body, and most importantly, produce the massive amounts of digestive enzymes necessary to extract nutrients from food in order for the body to benefit from its intake. Completely digesting the average meal, from the time the food enters the body until the waste leaves, can take hours or days depending on the type and quantity of the food (for example, pork is more difficult to digest then chicken, and chicken is more difficult to digest then watermelon). For all practical purposes though, if we are eating two to three meals a day, every day, then we are in a constant state of digestion. That is, every minute of every day our digestive system is working hard at breaking down foods, delivering nutrients, and expelling waste.

Meanwhile, all the other systems of the body, including the immune, respiratory, reproductive, cardiovascular, nervous, and muscular systems, must share the remaining 20 to 40 percent of the body's energy. Isn't that amazing? The digestive system consumes as much as four times more energy than all other systems combined.

Now imagine that something is amiss in one of the other systems in your body. The body is capable of handling the problem, but it requires additional energy to do so. Where does that additional energy come from? It is "stolen" from other systems, and most likely will affect the digestive system. (This is a very simplistic way of explaining a very complex system, but it makes the point.) This is why digestive symptoms are often the first clue that something is wrong with our bodies. It's possible that when we suddenly start experiencing indigestion, heartburn, acid reflux, gas, food cravings, bloating, and other digestive problems that the real culprit is something else entirely. For example, energy that could be used to balance the acid level in the stomach or produce digestive enzymes is being used elsewhere. Most people give little thought to the connection between their digestion and their overall health, but the two are inescapably intertwined (similar to the concept in Chinese medicine of yin and yang). And if we ignore these signs that something in the body is amiss, we set ourselves up for much more serious health issues down the road.

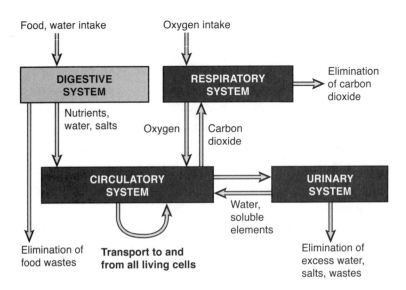

The digestive system links to all other systems in the body.

This is one of the reasons that the most obvious use of enzymes to overcome a health issue or symptom is to use them to enhance digestion. Whether the purpose is to improve a direct digestive problem or just free up energy for the body to use elsewhere, enzymes directly improve digestion by helping your body break down the food you consume. Understanding the digestive process is an important element of understanding how digestive enzymes can be so beneficial to your health.

THE DIGESTIVE PROCESS

Digestion begins in the mouth where the act of chewing breaks down and grinds food into smaller pieces to be swallowed. Think of the mouth as a food processor where mixing and grinding takes place. Three different types of amylase are secreted in the mouth to digest the carbohydrates we eat. The amylase is mixed with food when we chew, so it can begin working immediately. This is why it is so important to take the time to chew food well. The longer and better we chew, the more amylase we introduce to the food in our mouth.

When we swallow the food, it travels down the esophagus to the stomach. There are two sections of the stomach. The cardiac (upper) section is the first stop for the food we swallow. Though nothing is secreted in the cardiac section, this is where the majority of carbohydrate digestion occurs as the amylase from our saliva continues its work. The cardiac section is often called the food enzyme section of the stomach, since any active enzymes in the food we've eaten will also help partially digest the food. This will be discussed much more in the section on diet later in the chapter.

After about thirty to forty-five minutes in the cardiac section, the food enters the pyloric section or the lower stomach. Pepsin and hydrochloric acid (HCL) are secreted here to begin digesting proteins. The amount of protein consumed and the efficiency of the individual's digestive system will dictate the length of time the food remains in this portion of the stomach, but it's typically about two hours. Hydrochloric acid, pepsin, and muscular movement produce a thoroughly mixed, watery solution called chyme, which then leaves the stomach for the small intestine.

The Digestive System

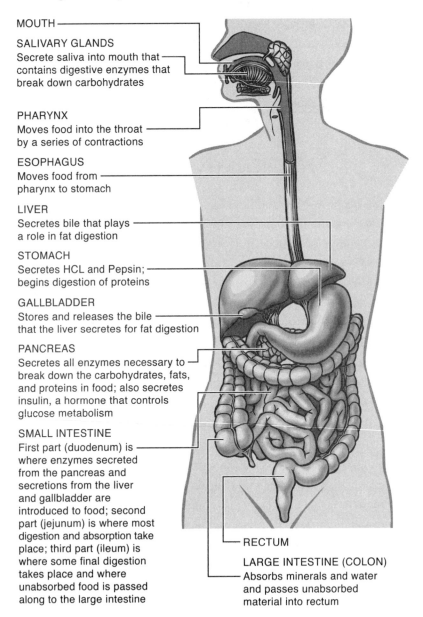

MOUTH

SALIVARY GLANDS
Secrete saliva into mouth that
contains digestive enzymes that
break down carbohydrates

PHARYNX
Moves food into the throat
by a series of contractions

ESOPHAGUS
Moves food from
pharynx to stomach

LIVER
Secretes bile that plays
a role in fat digestion

STOMACH
Secretes HCL and Pepsin;
begins digestion of proteins

GALLBLADDER
Stores and releases the bile
that the liver secretes for fat digestion

PANCREAS
Secretes all enzymes necessary to
break down the carbohydrates, fats,
and proteins in food; also secretes
insulin, a hormone that controls
glucose metabolism

SMALL INTESTINE
First part (duodenum) is
where enzymes secreted
from the pancreas and
secretions from the liver
and gallbladder are
introduced to food; second
part (jejunum) is where most
digestion and absorption take
place; third part (ileum) is
where some final digestion
takes place and where
unabsorbed food is passed
along to the large intestine

RECTUM

LARGE INTESTINE (COLON)
Absorbs minerals and water
and passes unabsorbed
material into rectum

When the chyme enters the small intestine, lipase secreted from the pancreas and bile secreted from the gallbladder assist with fat digestion. Acid from the stomach is also neutralized by secretions from the pancreas. It is at this point that the body takes a type of inventory of what we have eaten and what has been digested so far. Based on this information, it then determines the additional enzymes needed to finish the process. This is known as the law of adaptive secretion, by which the body only manufactures the amount of enzymes needed to process the carbohydrates, proteins, and fats that have reached this point undigested (Howell, 64–67). The pancreas will then manufacture and secrete the enzymes as needed. Note that this is a key way in which a healthy diet and digestive enzyme supplements can help the body. If the food reaches this point and has already been well digested, the body will not have to produce higher quantities of enzymes to continue to break the foods down in order to benefit from the nutrients.

Once through the small intestine (which is approximately twenty-three feet in length), the food finally enters the large intestine. This organ is basically responsible for absorbing water and electrolytes. Much of this process is the body reabsorbing what it has provided in the way of gastric juices. The large intestine is also home to a number (possibly hundreds) of different kinds of bacteria that live off of some of the foods (primarily fibrous foods) that have made it this far without being digested. As a byproduct of their metabolism, these beneficial bacteria make some of the vitamins we need and limit the growth of bad bacteria that can cause disease (see chapter 3). Once the large intestine has extracted these liquids and vitamins, the waste is eliminated.

FOOD ENZYMES AND DIET

The cells in plants are similar to those in both humans and animals: they need enzymes to survive. When we pick an apple off a tree, we have removed it from the branch, disconnecting it from its source of life. If the apple goes straight from the tree to our mouth, the naturally occurring enzymes in the apple will aid our digestive system. The enzymes that were once instrumental in cellular biochemical reactions necessary for the growth of the apple will be released as we chew and as the amylases in our saliva work to begin breaking down the cells of the apple. Those released enzymes can now contribute to the digestion of the apple in the cardiac (upper) section of the stomach.

We've all seen the physical evidence of these enzymes at work. I'm sure you've observed an apple going bad because it sat in the kitchen fruit bowl too long. You didn't eat it, so it ate itself. It deteriorated in front of your eyes. The enzymes within that apple became active in a digestive manner, and the result is a spoiled apple. If you want to speed up that process in a fresh apple, simply damage the apple in any way. The soft spots on apples are damaged areas where enzymes are particularly active (as they have been released from within the apple's cells) and the apple is being digested. When we chew the apple, we are literally speeding up the reaction we have watched in our kitchen fruit bowl. Add to this the 98-degree temperature inside our mouths, the naturally occurring amylases in our saliva, and the water contained in the apple, and you now have an environment perfectly suited to induce the greatest food enzyme activity possible. The enzymes that once assisted in keeping the apple alive now serve as digestive enzymes, and they take the burden of digestion off our body. The pancreas will still secrete enzymes to assist in the delivery of the nutrients from the apple to our cells, but far fewer are needed than if the apple had no active enzymes.

All raw vegetables and fruits contain the necessary active enzymes to break down the proteins, fats, and carbohydrates in those particular foods, lessening the burden on our digestive systems. However, raw food manifests only enough enzymes to digest itself, not enough to be stored in the body for later use or to assist in breaking down other foods consumed with it that may be void of enzymes. When we cook and process food, we denature the enzymes that occur naturally in the living organism, so they are no longer helpful in the digestive process. If we put that same apple in an apple pie or in apple sauce, the enzymes in it would be of no use to us digestively. When we eat cooked apples, the digestive system has to produce all of the enzymes needed to digest the cooked food.

THE DIETARY KEYS TO UNLOCKING GOOD HEALTH

So to lessen the burden on the digestive system and release potential energy for optimal functioning of all of the other systems, what is the ideal diet? Ideally, we would eat nutritionally healthy raw foods frequently and in small quantities. We would also limit calorie intake to under two thousand calories a day. Additionally, we would fast regularly to cleanse our digestive system and simultaneously give it a break. Each of these recommendations in its own way reduces the energy requirement of digesting food and as a result returns to the body the vital energy it needs to keep metabolic energy high enough to efficiently produce the metabolic enzymes needed to maintain optimal health. For example, restricting calories has been credited with increasing longevity, fasting has been credited with reversing disease, and eating raw food is associated with disease prevention (see appendix C). The fact is, though, most people will simply not follow the diet deemed "ideal." So let's discuss the *nearly* ideal diet.

The nearly ideal diet is a compromise, a combination of raw food, optimal calorie intake, occasional fasting, and digestive enzyme supplements. The key is making healthy decisions and choices. You decide what works for you, what you can live with, and where you will make tradeoffs when necessary; nothing more, nothing less. The good news is that when the decisions we make are less than ideal, we can make changes in something we don't mind sacrificing to keep the nearly ideal diet in balance. Note that you may want to consult a health care professional before making dramatic changes in your diet.

Let's look at this nearly ideal diet for Susan, who is in relatively good health. Susan is thirty-eight years old, not more than fifteen pounds overweight, exercises fairly regularly, and eats healthy foods most of the time, but she wants to make some changes to increase her energy, lose those extra pounds, and extend her life span and her health.

All Susan needs to do is

- Reduce the size of her meals by 25 percent, possibly adding more healthy (preferably raw) snacks to ensure that she is getting the right amount of calories
- Make at least one meal a day raw foods only
- Take a high-potency digestive enzyme with each meal
- Fast by eating raw food only, for at least five days, once every three months

Does that sound very difficult? The dividends it pays are truly amazing. The benefits to the average person include weight reduction (to your ideal, healthy weight), greater energy, reduced food cravings, more restful sleep, increased mental clarity, and most importantly a long-term improvement in your health and an extension of your life span.

The beauty of these recommendations is that if you fail in one of the four suggestions, you can modify another. If you have trouble eating a raw food meal every day, then you can increase the amount of digestive enzymes, reduce the meal size more than 25 percent and eat more frequently (lessening the intensity of the bursts of energy your body has to use to digest large meals), or fast every two months instead of every three months. The reason the nearly ideal diet is so adjustable is that every recommendation listed above contributes in a slightly different way to resting the digestive system and allowing the body to benefit from the additional energy.

These recommendations apply even when—especially when—we're sick. The more energy you can free up for the body to overcome a health issue, the better your chances of overcoming that issue. When we're feeling sick, although we might not have an appetite, we feel compelled to eat. And often we eat "comfort foods" to make us feel better, if only psychologically. But what our bodies really need when we're sick is a rest of the digestive system to free up that extra energy we need to get well. I am not suggesting we should refrain from eating when we're sick, but we need to consider eating foods that require little effort from the digestive system, and ones that are high in nutrition. Freshly juiced fruits and vegetables would be a great choice during times of illness. Fasting, eating raw foods, and restricting calories can also promote healing, increasing metabolic energy by reducing the demand for digestive energy. (Please note that the recommendations in this book are in no way intended to replace recommendations or advice from physicians or other health care providers. They are intended to support your path to optimal health. If you suspect you have a medical problem, I urge you to seek medical attention from a competent health care provider.)

Understanding the role of enzymes in digestion and health is so important it deserves a review. So to recap:

The first step in improving our overall health should always be to address digestion. Whether you're in a health crisis or just want to live a healthier life, this is where you must start. Ignoring this recommendation is like trying to hike up a mountain in flip-flops: it can be done, but it's not easy. You have to start with the basics.

If you want to stay healthy or get healthy you need to free up as much digestive energy as you can spare. This will help ensure all of the other systems of the body have the energy they need to function properly. Fasting, restricting calories, eating more raw food, or taking high-potency plant-based digestive enzymes at every meal can facilitate this. This is probably the single most effective approach you can take to maintain or regain health.

Though plant-based or animal-sourced enzymes may be used to treat digestive issues, the plant-based enzymes will provide the most digestive support. If the pancreas is inflamed, sluggish, or diseased, animal-sourced enzymes should be combined with plant-based enzymes as a regular part of a regimen. The animal-sourced enzymes will fortify the pancreas, while the plant-based enzymes will literally break down the food eaten.

In the next chapter, I discuss the importance of maintaining and promoting balance within other systems of the body. By maintaining this delicate balance of immune function, microflora in the intestinal tract, and the proper pH of the digestive system, you will be well on your way to that new path leading to additional energy, vitality, and health.

CHAPTER THREE
MAINTAINING THE DELICATE BALANCE

Enzymes relate directly to the working of the immune system, and though enzyme supplements have been shown to improve overall health, more needs to be done; balance must be achieved. There are three key areas of possible imbalance in the body that can affect the production of digestive and metabolic enzymes, cause one or more health crises, and potentially shorten our life span—immune system imbalances, pH imbalances, and bacterial (or microflora) imbalances. As mentioned in chapter 1, disease is essentially an imbalance that the body cannot correct due to the demand placed upon it. Though the health crisis may ultimately be the result of an enzyme deficiency, there are contributing factors that we do well to consider. The sooner we recognize the symptoms of imbalances and treat them, the sooner we will be on the path to good health, higher energy, and a longer life.

Please note that the recommendations in this book are in no way intended to replace recommendations or advice from physicians or other health care providers. They are intended to support your path to optimal health. If you suspect you have a medical problem, I urge you to seek medical attention from a competent health care provider.

MAINTAINING BALANCE WITHIN THE IMMUNE SYSTEM

The immune system is a whole-body network of cells and organs that, when working as intended, defends the body against attacks from "foreign" invaders. These invaders include bacteria, viruses, parasites, and fungi. There are times, however, when the immune system becomes either overactive or underactive. When it is underactive, we become vulnerable to many different diseases; when it is overactive, the immune system can begin to attack the body's own vital organs, tissue, and cells (this is usually called an autoimmune disease). Enzymes can help our bodies overcome or survive these imbalances.

AUTOIMMUNE DISEASES

Autoimmune diseases occur when the immune system's recognition apparatus breaks down, and the body begins to manufacture antibodies and T cells directed against its own cells and organs. This results in a variety of chronic, disabling illnesses. For instance, an antibody known as the rheumatoid factor is common in people with rheumatoid arthritis. According to the U.S. Department of Health and Human Services, autoimmune diseases collectively affect 14.7 to 23.5 million people, and the incidence is rising (January 2003).

Though few agree on the causes of autoimmune diseases, there are some popular theories. One has to do with the production of immune complexes when immune responses are trying to overcome a threat. Once the threat is gone, the immune complexes may settle in tissue and joints, signaling the immune system to act upon those specific areas. Another theory is that inflammation on a microscopic level produces this same immune reaction. Still other theories place the blame on viruses, bacteria, toxins, or heavy metals. What all of these theories have in common is the idea that the immune system is looking for something it cannot find, something that does not exist or exists for no apparent reason (something that poses no real threat). Another common link is that protease can act on many of the elements that are suspected causes of the immune system attacking the body.

For instance, heavy metals, such as lead and mercury, exert their poisoning effect by binding to groups of proteins, including vital enzymes. Once they bind to a functional enzyme, they denature it, inhibit it, or both. This interaction of heavy metals with proteins can lead to degenerating diseases, nerve damage, or even death. Some clinical observations have shown that when proteases are taken in large amounts, heavy metal concentrations decrease significantly in the blood.

ALLERGIES

When the immune system malfunctions, it can unleash a torrent of disorders and diseases. One of the most familiar is an allergic response. Allergies such as hay fever and hives are related to a specific type of antibody known as IgE. The first time an allergy-prone person is exposed to an allergen—for example, grass pollen—the individual's B cells make large amounts of the grass pollen-specific IgE antibody. These IgE molecules attach to histamine-containing cells known as mast cells, which are plentiful in the lungs, skin, tongue, and linings of the nose and gastrointestinal tract. The next time this person encounters grass pollen, the IgE-primed mast cell releases powerful chemicals (histamine) that cause the wheezing, sneezing, and other symptoms of an allergic reaction. This is the body's defense system trying to rid the body of a perceived threat. Enzymes may assist by either helping the body recognize the intruder as nonharmful or by inhibiting the reaction by breaking down histamine.

So immune imbalances can contribute in a large way to serious illness. It is imperative to maintain balance in this system, and enzyme supplementation, in particular protease supplementation, can do much to achieve the needed balance (see appendix C).

THE IMPORTANCE OF PROPER pH BALANCE

Enzyme supplements help balance the immune system, but they can't solve all the body's problems, and some health issues can affect how well they work and how much they benefit our health. One such example is the body's pH balance.

The body must maintain a specific acid-alkaline balance to survive. This balance is measured in terms of pH. The term "pH," which actually stands for potential of hydrogen (or as a good friend of mine, Dr. Robert Striesfeld, says, "pH stands for potential of health"), is defined by a scale from 0 to 14 that assigns a number to indicate acidity and alkalinity. The lower the pH number, the more acid it is. The higher the number, the more alkaline it is. For example, a pH of 3 is more acidic than a pH of 5. A pH of 9 is more alkaline than a pH of 6. A pH of 7 is neutral.

Maintaining proper pH is much more critical in certain parts of the body than others. For instance, pH within the blood cannot vary much at all or death will quickly follow. On the other hand, the digestive system should maintain a specific acid-alkaline balance, but it can vary widely. It is out of balance more often than not in most adults. This is a good example of the body's ability to prioritize. Although it will do all it can to maintain the specific pH required in the blood, the body is often unable to meet the same specifications throughout the digestive tract. If it did, some other part of the body (perhaps a more critical organ or system) may be adversely affected due to neglect.

For humans, a normal pH of all tissues and fluids of the body (except the stomach) is slightly alkaline. All other organs and fluids will fluctuate in their pH range in order to keep the blood at a strict pH between 7.35 and 7.45. Too much acidity or alkalinity in the body can have far-reaching consequences. For example, if the blood becomes too acidic

- It takes some of the alkaline-forming elements from the enzymes in the small intestine to stay balanced. The small intestine then becomes too acidic to digest foods optimally. The pancreas, gallbladder, and liver are then forced to make up for this deficiency in order to metabolize foods properly. This has a direct bearing on metabolic enzyme production and metabolic energy, which results in lowered immune function, fatigue, hormonal imbalances, absorption and digestive problems, and many other problems as well.

- Calcium is leeched from the bones, since it is the most alkaline of the minerals. This occurs as the body struggles to maintain the homeostasis of the blood pH. This condition can lead to reduced absorption of supplemental minerals and bone density problems, including osteoporosis.

- Insulin levels increase and fat is stored instead of being metabolized. This is due to the body mimicking what happens when malnutrition or starvation sets in. Interestingly, the body increases in acidity when malnourished; as a safety mechanism, insulin is overproduced, so that all available calories are stored as fat for future use. As a result, weight gain is common and weight loss becomes more difficult.

- Electrolyte imbalances occur, which have a direct bearing on the fluid transport system. Electrolytes are important since they maintain the electrical voltage existing around all cells, especially critical around the cells of the heart, nervous system, and muscles.

Similar problems may occur if the body becomes too alkaline, though this is much less likely. Overall the symptoms that might occur if the pH in the body is out of balance include but are not limited to acid reflux, indigestion, weight gain, difficulty losing weight, poor metabolism, mineral deficiencies, constipation, fatigue, brain fog, frequent urination, hypoglycemia, hormonal imbalances, and sore muscles.

Some of the factors that contribute to this imbalance include stress, environmental pollution, too little or too much exercise, and the most important factor, diet. The more acid-forming foods we eat, the more acidic we become. The more alkaline-forming foods we eat, the more alkaline we become. Generally speaking, fruits and vegetables are more alkaline-forming, while meats, sugar, caffeine, beans, dairy, and grains are more acid forming.

Notice the term "generally speaking" in the previous sentence. Gabriel Cousens, in *Conscious Eating*, mentions the complexity of this topic. His research has shown that about 30 percent of the people he counseled responded exactly opposite to this claim. In other words, the fruits and vegetables they ate made them *more* acidic. So we must be willing to take the time to determine individually what foods will work best for *us*.

Regardless of the cause, it is obvious that maintaining the proper pH in the blood, digestive tract, tissues, and fluids is essential in order to support optimal health.

DETERMINING YOUR pH

One of the best ways to determine whether or not you are maintaining a proper pH is to test your urine (usually using pH paper, sold in health food stores). This is an accurate way to almost directly assess the pH of your body, because the kidneys are the main organ system that balances the pH of the body. If we become too acidic, our kidneys will eliminate and remove acid through the urine. If we are too alkaline, the same is true, it will show in the urine. This is part of the regulation mechanism of the body and contributes to keeping blood alkalinity in balance. The urine will always reflect what the body is getting rid of. Urine, then, is an excellent indicator to determine whether or not we are maintaining a proper pH balance.

Although many people believe that the best time to test urine pH is the first thing in the morning, it is better to test pH repeatedly over a period of twenty-four hours. The morning pH of the urine will almost always be the most acidic of the day, since it is at night that we detoxify and the kidneys remove a lot of acid. It is much more accurate to track pH throughout the day and then calculate the average. In order to optimally benefit from this exercise, you should also keep a log of the foods consumed. This will help quickly determine which foods and drinks contribute to your pH levels. Then you will be able to make adjustments to stay in balance through dietary changes.

The optimal urine pH is between 6 and 7. If your average is below 6, you are too acidic. If your average is above 7, you are too alkaline. In either case you should immediately consider lifestyle changes to support the proper pH for your body.

Saliva is also often recommended as a good indicator of pH balance. Nevertheless, this method is very unreliable. Most people test alkaline when testing their saliva alone, while most people test acidic when testing only their urine. The fact is that when a person's saliva tests acidic, it indicates an extreme imbalance, but saliva testing as alkaline is common even if a person is too acidic. Most experts agree that the pH of saliva is an indicator of alkaline reserve. (The body does not create alkalinity; rather it has an alkaline mineral reserve based on the dietary intake of alkaline foods.) Saliva naturally contains minerals. When those minerals are not present, then there is a problem; this indicates a depleted alkaline reserve or a mineral deficiency.

If you do decide to go the saliva route, here are some helpful guidelines: The healthy pH of saliva tested first thing in the morning or on an empty stomach is between 6.2 and 7.2. After a meal it should become even more alkaline. One theory is that if the pH of the saliva is between 5.8 and 6.2, the body is too acidic with little alkaline reserve left. If the morning pH is below 5.8 with no rise after meals, there is no alkaline reserve left and the body is extremely acidic.

TREATING A pH IMBALANCE

There are a number of products sold in health food stores that may help balance pH, but caution should be exercised. In my opinion most products formulated to help raise alkalinity are too alkaline. I have tested some of the most popular products sold for this purpose and the majority of products average 10 on the pH scale. The most alkaline part of the digestive system, meanwhile, is the small intestine, which averages 8 on the pH scale. The problem with putting something so alkaline in your gut is that it neutralizes stomach acid. The stomach averages between 2 and 3 on the pH scale. When stomach acid is neutralized, the body will work overtime trying to maintain the naturally acid environment of the stomach. This mechanism creates a demand to constantly produce more acid, which is obviously counterproductive when the goal is to become more alkaline.

This common response is why the person who consumes "antacids" for heartburn will need more and more as time goes on. Whereas at first a couple tablets did the trick, soon at least five or six are required for any relief at all. This vicious cycle continues until the person begins taking prescription H2 blockers or proton pump inhibitors that literally shut off the acid faucet. Of course, this has other detrimental consequences, including poor protein digestion, ulcers, and gas, to name just a few.

The solution to the dilemma is actually quite simple. In order to raise alkalinity safely, you should take a product that does not exceed the natural pH of the small intestine and does not upset the acidity of the stomach. This can be achieved by using a formula that maintains a pH of 8 and is enteric coated. This protects the capsule or tablet from breaking down in the naturally acidic environment of the stomach and instead releases the ingredients in the small intestine, where they belong. There the ingredients can restore balance to this vital section of the intestinal tract and ultimately to the whole body. The beauty of this kind of formula is that if the person taking it is too alkaline (meaning the pH of the small intestine is above 8) the same formula can contribute to reducing alkalinity. This method truly balances pH, rather than just raising alkalinity.

The only companies that I am aware of that go to such great lengths to create moderately alkaline, enteric-coated products are Enzymedica and Theramedix. The Enzymedica product is called pH Basic and the Theramedix product is called pHB. (More information on these companies is provided at the end of the next chapter.) Following are some of the ingredients active in such formulas.

- A mineral blend that consists of the same minerals often depleted in an acid environment and those that make up the electrolyte mineral ratio; these include potassium bicarbonate, sodium bicarbonate, and magnesium citrate

- An organic super food such as hydrilla, a type of green, which is naturally alkaline. Hydrilla is nature's most potent source of calcium, and one of the richest plant sources of many trace minerals and amino acids.

- An enzyme blend formulated to promote the absorption of the ingredients (the minerals, herbs, and greens)

- Marshmallow root and papaya leaf extract, to help soothe the common symptoms that are associated with high acidity

- A delivery system that bypasses the acid stomach and goes straight to the small intestine

In addition to a supplement designed to bring the pH back in balance, in order to maintain optimum pH balance, it is important to ensure proper digestion and assimilation of the foods you eat. One of the best ways to stay balanced is to take plant-based enzymes with every meal. These enzymes assist the body in breaking down and assimilating the nutrients in the foods you eat regardless of pH.

HELPFUL CHANGES

Diet is probably the most important change to make in creating a healthy lifestyle and maintaining proper pH. Avoid the overconsumption of meat, alcohol, soft drinks, caffeine, coffee, most nuts, eggs, vinegar, sauerkraut, ascorbic acid (vitamin C), pasteurized milk, cheese, white sugar, and medical drugs. Add additional servings of ripe fruit, vegetables, soybeans, bean sprouts, water, raw milk, onions, figs, carrots, beets, miso, and mineral supplements.

It also helps to reduce anxiety when possible and include moderate exercise in your daily regimen. Strenuous exercise can actually contribute to an acidic environment in the body because of the increased production of lactic acid. Though I am not suggesting that strenuous exercise is bad, if one is having difficulty achieving an acid–alkaline balance, it should be a consideration.

MICROFLORA BALANCE

Another often-ignored health threat that can affect your overall wellness and life span comes from bacteria. Bacteria are simple single-celled organisms that are found everywhere on earth. They are so prevalent that it is believed they are likely the most numerous type of organism on the planet. Though most bacteria are not harmful, we often think first of those bacteria that are, such as *Streptococcus*, which cause strep throat, *Staphylococcus*, the cause of "staph" infections, or *E. coli*, a common cause of food poisoning. But bacteria and other microflora have far more complex and beneficial roles.

Within our body and in particular within our intestinal tract, bacteria play a vital role in overall health. The condition and function of the trillions of bacteria or microflora in our gastrointestinal tract are essential to our well-being. By some estimates there are more than five hundred species of bacteria in our intestinal tract alone. They represent between 30 percent and 50 percent of the total weight of the contents of the intestinal tract. We have a symbiotic relationship with these microflora; they protect against the overgrowth of pathogenic organisms, assist in the digestion of fiber and lactose, produce enzymes, and manufacture B vitamins. In turn, we give these friendly bacteria a place to live and food to prosper.

If the population of good microflora diminishes to the point where many of these beneficial actions cease, opportunistic "bad" organisms can take their place and wreak havoc on the body. One such opportunistic yeast is called *Candida albicans*. When the opportunity arises, this yeast, which normally resides in the colon in relatively small numbers, can overgrow. In the overgrowth state it can actually form "roots" that burrow through the intestinal lining and strip the colon of all of its beneficial microflora. This can lead to irritable bowel syndrome (IBS), chronic yeast infections, skin problems, immune disorders, and numerous digestive issues.

The cause of this imbalance of bacteria is most often the administration of antibiotics, which decreases metabolic activities within the colonies. Antibiotics do not discriminate; in their presence all bacteria die, the good with the bad. Birth control pills, cortisone, and a poor diet may increase the possibility of a *Candida* overgrowth. To maintain or reestablish a healthy balance, probiotics may be the most natural, safe, and commonsense approach. A probiotic is the exact opposite of an antibiotic; it is made up of beneficial bacteria and can recolonize the digestive tract to reestablish balance.

Your body's microflora also have several connections to enzymes that make them important:

- Like enzymes, microflora are essential for good digestion.
- Microflora produce enzymes (cellulase, lactase, protease, and amylase) to complete digestion and synergize with other enzymes in support of the immune system.
- Like enzymes, microflora are instrumental in protecting us from invading bacteria and viruses.

Probiotics are a great adjunct to supplemental enzymes, since enzymes taken as a supplement eventually become inactive due to the exhaustion of energy; they wear out. The enzymes in a supplement have a life of three to eight hours, whereas probiotics, once established in the intestinal tract, can colonize and grow, continuing to provide benefits for long periods of time. Probiotics reintroduce good bacteria to live in the gut, colonize, and create more enzymes. But when the microflora of the intestines are out of balance, enzyme therapy to support the digestive process is more important than ever.

WHAT TO LOOK FOR IN A GOOD PROBIOTIC

When it comes to picking a probiotic there are many choices. The choice is often confusing, though, because of the number of different bacteria strains available, the process of manufacturing, and the way companies label their products. Today you can find products containing one strain of bacteria and others with twenty strains. The most common are *Lactobacillus acidophilus* and *L. bifidus;* these are supported by more research and have been in use longer than any of the other choices. The problem with these strains is that they are not very hardy; they die rather easily from exposure to heat, acid, and air, so the potency at time of consumption has been shown to be suspect.

Many companies that sell products with these microflora as the main ingredients will often state that the number of CFUs (colony forming units) contained in the capsule are "at time of manufacture." This is basically telling the customer that by the time they consume the product there is no telling exactly how many of these sensitive bacteria will be alive, which is one of the reasons that so much scrutiny has been placed on these products. Often fewer than half of the probiotic products tested will meet their label claim. For this reason I always recommend that you look for a probiotic that guarantees potency at the *time of consumption.*

You should also look for a supplement that has a delivery system that ensures the friendly bacteria will survive the trip. Some bacteria strains have been shown to survive the acid environment of the stomach, such as *Bacillus subtillus* and *Lactobacillus F-19*, but most cannot. For the strains that have difficulty surviving, it is best to deliver them in an enteric-coated capsule that will protect the sensitive bacteria from the stomach acid, delivering it safely to the intestinal tract.

Some of the more common strains you will find (in addition to *L. acidophilus* and *L. bifidus*) include *Lactobacillus casei, Lactobacillus bulgaris, Bacillus subtillus, Lactobacillus plantarum, Lactobacillus rhamnosus, Lactobacillus salivarius, Lactobacillus longum, Lactobacillus lactis* and *Lactobacillus F-19*.

Obviously, unless you have studied probiotics and bacteria, these strains may not mean anything you. The following is a listing of the eight strains that I believe are the most noteworthy, along with some descriptions from the studies that investigate their benefit.

LACTOBACILLUS ACIDOPHILUS

- "*Lactobacillus acidophilus* helps to control diarrhea and reduce bad cholesterol by converting it to coprostanol and enabling its elimination. It helps in the reduction of lactose intolerance and in the control of *Candida* overgrowth, it protects the gastrointestinal tract, and it strengthens the immune system."[1]

- "For example, the breakdown of food by *L. acidophilus* leads to production of lactic acid, hydrogen peroxide, and other byproducts that make the environment hostile for undesired organisms. *L. acidophilus* also produces lactase, the enzyme that breaks down milk sugar (lactose) into simple sugars. People who are lactose intolerant do not produce this enzyme. For this reason, *L. acidophilus* supplements may be beneficial for these individuals."[2]

LACTOBACILLUS CASEI

- "*Lactobacillus casei* is effective in the treatment of intestinal infections. It inhibits tumors in mice and increases immunity in humans against bacterial and viral infections. *L. casei* encourages proper gastrointestinal function and elimination and maintains the balance of the gastrointestinal terrain."[3]

- "Oral administration of *Lactobacillus casei* has been found to enhance innate immunity by stimulating the activity of . . . NK cells. The ability to switch mucosal immune responses . . . with probiotic bacteria provides a strategy for treatment of allergic disorders."[4]

LACTOBACILLUS BULGARICUS

- "*Lactobacillus bulgaricus* does not colonize in the intestinal tract, is fast growing, and produces lactic acid; it thus promotes the growth of beneficial bacteria that establish a balanced gastrointestinal tract environment. It contributes to digestion, lactose tolerance, the reduction of cholesterol, and the control of intestinal infections and it also enhances immunity."[5]

- Beneficial *L. bulgaricus* colonies "form a hostile environment for pathogenic (disease-causing) germs and play a major detoxification role in removing potentially harmful germs that travel through the gastrointestinal (GI) tract. This cleansing activity also helps sweep metabolic waste and chemical toxins from the body. *L. bulgaricus* helps in correcting the condition of either constipation or diarrhea by significantly influencing the peristaltic action of the GI tract. Chronic, persistent diarrhea is less common in infants fed yogurt containing *L. bulgaricus* compared to milk fed infants."[6]

LACTOBACILLUS PLANTARUM

- "*Lactobacillus plantarum* produces lactic acid, inhibits the growth of gastrointestinal tract pathogens, and prevents flatulence. One strain of the *L. plantarum* species has been tested clinically for its effect on irritable bowel syndrome (IBS). In both studies, subjects showed a decrease in IBS symptoms and reduced pain."[7]

- "*L. plantarum* appears to help preserve nutrients such as omega-3 fatty acids, but also increase their content. *L. plantarum* has also demonstrated the ability to reduce and eliminate potentially pathogenic microorganisms both in vitro and in vivo."[8]

- "In a 4-week, double-blind, placebo-controlled trial of 60 individuals with IBS, probiotics treatment with *L. plantarum* reduced intestinal gas significantly."[9]

LACTOBACILLUS RHAMNOSUS

- "*Lactobacillus rhamnosus* provides mucosal support by adhering to the mucosal membrane, inhibiting fungal or bacterial vaginal infections, and preventing infection. *L. rhamnosus* . . . reduce the incidence of or lessen the severity of antibiotic-associated diarrhea."[10]

- "According to a recent study in 10 healthy adults, cellular immune response to intestinal microorganisms was enhanced following intake of *L. rhamnosus* GG for 5 weeks. This increased the response of peripheral T lymphocytes to intestinal bacteria and enhanced an inflammatory response by increasing the secretion of suppressive cytokines and decreasing secretion of pro-inflammatory cytokines."[11]

- "Administration of *L. rhamnosus* GG to pregnant mother weeks prior to delivery and to their newborn babies through 6 months of age led to a 50% decrease in the infants' incidence of recurring atopic eczema."[12]

LACTOBACILLUS SALIVARIUS

- "*Lactobacillus salivarius* prevents flatulence and inhibits intestinal putre-faction and the development of undesirable bacteria in the mouth and intestines. It is antibiotic resistant and therefore helps to prevent antibi-otic-induced diarrhea."[13]

- "*L. salivarius* is classified as a facultative bacterium, which means that it can survive and grow in both anaerobic (without oxygen) and aero-bic (with oxygen) environments, although its main effects take place in anaerobic conditions. One unique benefit of *L. salivarius* is its ability to help break down undigested protein and disengage the toxins produced by protein putrefactions. In one study, *L. salivarius* was able to produce a high amount of lactic acid and completely inhibit the growth of *H. pylori* in a mixed culture. *L. salivarius* was found to be a potentially effective probiotic against *H. pylori*."[14]

BACILLUS SUBTILIS

- This bacterium is the source of nattokinase, the enzyme that has been discovered to support cardiovascular health and balance blood viscosity. It is one of the most studied strains in the world and has been shown to normalize intestinal microflora balance.

- *B. subtilis* is able to secrete large amounts of extracellular enzymes, includ-ing a-amylase, arabinase, cellulase, dextranase, levansucrase, maltase, alka-line protease, neutral protease, B. glucanase, DNase, and various enzymes with N. acetylmuramidase activity. *B. subtilis* is able to grow and exert a positive metabolic effect in different habitats, including soil and the GI tract of animals and man. It is one of the most important anti-diarrhea microorganisms used in human medicine, used primarily for the therapy and prophylaxis of intestinal disorders resulting from antibiotic therapy.[15]

LACTOBACILLUS F19

- *Lactobacillus F-19* is a member of the *Lactobacillus acidophilus* paracasei species. It is well tolerated by infants, adults, and the elderly, adheres to the colon, and persists in the GI tract. It has also been shown to increase lac-tic acid bacteria in the GI microflora after eight weeks of consumption.

- *Lactobacillus F-19* is an emerging probiotic that has a proven ability to survive gastric transit. It not only persists in the colonic environment of humans, but it also increases other lactic acid bacteria in the GI microflora.[16]

A WORD ABOUT PROTEASE AND PROBIOTICS

There has been some recent concern that protease taken with probiotics kills both the probiotics consumed orally and the microflora that are already a part of the intestinal ecosystem. This idea is based on the simplistic understanding that protease breaks down protein. Though this is true, it is incomplete.

Plant-based proteases (from aspergillus) have the ability to break down a fairly wide range of proteins in a reasonably wide pH. However, they do not break down all proteins. In order for these proteases to break down proteins, at least one of the following must be met: The protein must be dead, as in the case when we eat protein; the protein must be damaged; the protein must be tagged for removal by the immune system. If these plant-based proteins did indeed break down all proteins, then all red blood cells, white blood cells, muscle tissues, stomach lining, arteries, other enzymes, and practically every other tissue of the body would be in danger.

Another point to consider is the content of the probiotics themselves. They are bacterial organisms, full of enzymes, including proteases. Why don't the proteases in the probiotic kill the cell? The answer is obvious: the protease in bacteria is specific and does not digest the living protein found in the bacteria itself.

Enzymes are helpful in addressing a wide range of issues in the body, but when any one system is out of balance, they are especially important. Any imbalance in the body puts strain on all of the other systems as the body attempts to compensate. Using enzymes digestively and therapeutically will support the body's efforts to get back in balance.

STUDIES:

1. Rosell, J. M.; Brochu, E.; Vezina C. et al. Rosell Institute Inc, unpublished data, 1997. Harmsen, H. J.; Wildeboer-Veloo, A. C.; Raangs, G. C. et al. "Analysis of intestinal flora development in breast-fed and formula-fed infants by using molecular identification and detection methods." *J Pediatr Gastroenterol Nutr.* 30 (2000): 61–67.

2. Alvarez-Olmos, M. I.; Oberhelman, R. A. "Probiotic agents and infectious diseases: a modern perspective on a traditional therapy." Clin Infect Dis. 32 (11) (Jun 1, 2001): 1567–76. Cunningham-Rundles, S.; Ahrne, S.; Bengmark S. et al. "Probiotics and immune response." *Am J Gastroenterol* 95 (1 Suppl) (Jan. 200): S22–5.

3. The Burton Goldberg Group. *Alternative Medicine: The Definitive Guide.* (Fife, WA: Future Medicine Publishing, Inc., 1995). Institute for Functional Medicine, Inc. *Clinical Nutrition: A Functional Approach.* Gig Harbor, WA: The Institute for Functional Medicine; 1999.

4. Matsuzaki T., Chin J. "Modulating immune responses with probiotic bacteria." *Immunology and Cell Biology* v.78, no. 1 (February 2000): 67–73(7).

5. Institute for Functional Medicine, Inc. *Clinical Nutrition: A Functional Approach.* Gig Harbor, WA: The Institute for Functional Medicine, 1999. Jarnason, I.; Williams, P.; Smethurst, P. et al. "Effect of non-steroidal anti-inflammatory drugs and prostaglandins on the permeability of the human small intestine." *Gut* 27 (1986): 1292–1297.

6. Bergogne-Berezin, E. "Treatment and prevention of antibiotic associated diarrhea." *Int J Antimicrob Agents.* 16(4) (2000 Dec):521–6. Bryant, M. "The shift to probiotics." *The Journal of Alternative Medicine* 2 (1986): 6–9. Tejada-Simon, M. "Proinflammatory cytokine and nitric oxide induction in murine macrophages by cell wall and cytoplasmic extracts of lactic acid bacteria." Department of Food Science and Human Nutrition, Michigan State University, 1999.

7. Niedzielin, K.; Kordecki, H.; Birkenfeld, B. "A controlled, double-blind, randomized study on the efficacy of *Lactobacillus plantarum* 299V in patients with irritable bowel syndrome." *Eur J Gastroenterol Hepatol.* 13(10) (Oct. 2001): 1143–7. Nobaek, S; Johansson, ML; Molin, G.; Ahrne, S.; Jeppsson, B. "Alteration of intestinal microflora is associated with reduction in abdominal bloating and pain in patients with irritable bowel syndrome." *Am J Gastroenterol.* 95(5) (May 2000): 1231–8.

8. Benmark, S. *Nutrition* 14, nos. 7–8 (July 1998): 585–94.

9. Nobaek, S.; Johansson, M. L.; Molin, G. et al. "Alteration of intestinal microflora is associated with reduction in abdominal bloating and pain in patients with irritable bowel syndrome." *Am J Gastroenterol.* 95 (2000): 1231–1238.

10. Heyman, M. J. *Am. Coll. Nutr.* 19 (2000): 137s.

11. Schultz, M.; Linde, H. J.; Lehn, N. et al. *J. Dairy Res.* 70 (2003): 165.

12. Kalliomaki, M.; Salminen, S.; Arvilommi, H. et al. *Lancet 357* (2001): 1076.

13. Rosell, J. M.; Brochu, E.; Vezina, C. et al., Rosell Institute Inc., unpublished data, 1997.

14. Aiba Y., Suzuki N., Kabir A. M., Takagi A., Koga Y. "Lactic acid-mediated suppression of *Helicobacter pylori* by the oral administration of *Lactobacillus salivarius* as a probiotic in a gnotobiotic murine model." *Am J Gastroenterol.* 93 (11) (Nov. 1998): 2097–101. Kabir, A.M. *Gut* 41, no. 1 (July 1997): 49–55.

15. Hosoi T., Ametani A., Kiuchi K., Kaminogawa K. "Improved growth and viability of lactobacilli in the presence of *Bacillus subtilis* (natto), catalase, or subtilisin." *Can. J. Microbiol./Rev. Can. Microbiol.* 46(10) (2000): 892–897. Mazza P. "The use of *Bacillus subtilis* as an antidiarrhoeal microorganism." *Boll Chim Farm.* 133(1) (1994 Jan): 3–18.

16. "*Lactobacillus Paracasei* subsp. paracasei F19: Survival, Ecology and Safety in the Human Intestinal Tract—A Survey of Feeding Studies within the PROBDEMO Project." Crittenden, R.; Saarela, M.; Mättö, J. et al. *Microbial Ecology in Health and Disease* 14 (1) supplement 3 (March 2002): 22–26. Bennet, R.; Nord, C. E.; Mättö, J. "Faecal recovery and absence of side effects in children given Lactobacillus F19 or placebo." Functional foods for EU-health in 2000, 4th Workshop, FAIR CT96-1028, PROBDEMO, VTT Symposium 198, Rovaniemi, Finland, 72. Miettinen, M; Voupio-Varkila, J.; and Varkila, K. "Production of human tumour necrosis factor alpha, interleukin-6 and interleukin-10 is induced by lactic acid bacteria." *Infection and Immunity* 64 (1996): 5403–5405. Salminen, S.; Laine, M.; von Wright, A. et al. "Development of selection criteria for probiotics strains to assess their potential in functional food. A Nordic and European approach." *Bioscience Microflora* 15 (1996): 61–67.

CHAPTER FOUR
SIMPLE ENZYME PROGRAMS FOR BETTER HEALTH

As you may have figured out by now, enzymes can be used in a variety of ways to treat a variety of health issues, or even just to help maintain our overall health and improve our longevity. Incorporating enzyme therapy into our lives is very easy to do, and I've developed a few standard programs that almost anyone can use to address common health concerns, without having to learn about every available enzyme supplement and how it might apply to you.

I'll begin this chapter with a brief discussion of the most common enzymes used in enzyme therapy and in enzyme blends you can purchase. Then I'll discuss how to determine if you're enzyme deficient and in what way, and offer recommendations for treating those deficiencies. Next, I'll present five simple enzyme therapy programs that will help you maintain your health in a way that meets your specific needs. I'll end the chapter with a discussion of what to look for when buying enzyme supplements and where to find them.

Before we delve into specific enzymes and enzyme therapy programs, I'd like to say a word about taking enzyme supplements. Throughout this chapter and the rest of the book, I've provided recommendations for various supplements to be taken with and between meals. The number of capsules to take varies with an individual's circumstances. For example, a person in excellent health with a strict diet that includes eating five times a day may only need one capsule of a digestive enzyme blend with each meal. On the other hand, an individual in poor health (undergoing a severe health crisis) who eats three large meals a day without doing any exercise may need two to three capsules with meals. Use your good judgment when deciding how many capsules to take, beginning with the recommendations as a starting point.

ENZYMES USED IN SUPPLEMENTS

There are new enzymes being discovered every day, but there are a few enzymes that are used commonly in therapy and supplements. I've outlined these enzymes in the "Enzymes and Their Uses" table, offering key information that will help you understand how they might benefit you. Use this table as a reference as you determine how you will incorporate enzyme therapy into your life.

ENZYMES AND THEIR USES

Enzyme	Category	Purpose	Unit of Measurement
Alpha-galactosidase	Carbohydrase	• Breaks down carbohydrates, such as raffinose and stachyose • Especially helpful with digestion of raw vegetables and beans	Galactosidase units (GALU)
Amylase	Carbohydrase	• Breaks down carbohydrates, such as starch and glycogen • Regulates histamine when taken on an empty stomach • Reduces food cravings • Increases blood sugar • Available from different sources and can be blended to increase potency	Dextrinizing units (DU) and Sanstedt Kneen Blish Units (SKB)

Enzyme	Category	Purpose	Unit of Measurement
Beta-glucanase	Carbohydrase	• Breaks down carbohydrates, especially glucan, a carbohydrate found in barley, oats, and wheat • Particularly beneficial as a digestive enzyme for people who have difficulty digesting grain-based products	Betaglucanase units (BGU)
Bromelain	Protease	• Breaks down protein • Most beneficial as an anti-inflammatory	Gelatin digesting units (GDU) and papain units (FCCPU)
Catalase	Protease	• Acts as an antioxidant by breaking down hydrogen peroxide into water and oxygen • One of the most potent antioxidants; found in nearly every cell of the body	Baker units
Cellulase	Carbohydrase	• Breaks down cellulose and chitin, a celluloselike fiber found in the cell wall of Candida (yeast) • Helps free nutrients in both fruits and vegetables because of its action on the cell wall • Available from different sources and can be blended to increase potency	Cellulase units (CU)
Glucoamylase	Carbohydrase	• Breaks down carbohydrates, specifically polysaccharides (long chains of carbohydrates) • Particularly beneficial as a digestive enzyme	Amygalactosidase units (AGU)
Hemicellulase	Carbohydrase	• Breaks down carbohydrates, especially polysaccharides found in plants • Particularly beneficial as a digestive enzyme for people who have difficulty digesting vegetable material	Hemicellulase units (HCU)
Invertase (sucrase)	Carbohydrase	• Breaks down carbohydrates, especially sucrose and maltose • Particularly beneficial as a digestive enzyme for people who are intolerant of sugars	Invertase active units (IAU)

Enzyme	Category	Purpose	Unit of Measurement
Lactase	Carbohydrase	• Breaks down lactose (milk sugar) • Used to treat lactose intolerance	Lactase units (LacU)
Lipase	Lipase	• Breaks down lipids and improves fat utilization • Helps reduce cholesterol • Supports weight loss • Supports hormone production • Supports gallbladder function • Available from different sources and can be blended to increase potency	FCCFIP (Food Chemical Codex Federation International Pharmaceutique) and lipase units (LU)
Maltase (diastase, malt diastase)	Carbohydrase	• Breaks down carbohydrates, especially malt and grain sugars and complex and simple sugars	Degrees of diastatic power (DP)
Mucolase	Protease	• Breaks down mucus • Helpful for congestion and sinus infections • Noncrystalline form of seaprose	Milligrams and mucolase units (MSU)
Nattokinase	Protease	• Breaks down fibrin, a clotting protein that forms in the blood after trauma or injury and as a result of viruses, fungi, and toxins in the blood • Used to treat cardiovascular issues, circulation issues, high blood pressure, slow tissue repair	Fibrinolytic units (FU)
Papain	Protease	• Breaks down protein • Most beneficial as an anti-inflammatory	Food Chemical Codex papain units (FCCPU)
Pectinase	Carbohydrase	• Breaks down carbohydrates, such as pectin, found in many fruits and vegetables	Apple juice depectinizing units (AJDU)
Phytase	Carbohydrase	• Breaks down carbohydrates, especially phytic acid, found in the leaves of plants • Helps with mineral absorption	Phytase units (PU)

Enzyme	Category	Purpose	Unit of Measurement
Protease	Protease	• Breaks down protein • Bonds with alpha 2-macro-globulin to support immune function when taken on an empty stomach • Reduces inflammation and increases circulation • Available from different sources and can be blended to increase potency	Hemoglobin units in a tyrosine base (HUT)
Seaprose	Protease	• Breaks down mucus • Helps with congestion and sinus infections • A crystalline (more concentrated) form of mucolase	Milligrams (mg)
Serratiopeptidase or serapeptase or serrapeptidase	Protease	• Anti-inflammatory	Measured in Serratio-peptidase Units (SU) (this is a relatively new enzyme and does not yet have an abbreviation; it will simply say "10,000 units" on the bottle)
Superoxide Dis-mutase (SOD)	Protease	• Antioxident • Protects cells from free radical damage	Milligrams (mg)
Xylanase	Carbohydrase	• A type of hemicellulase • Breaks down soluble fiber rather than insoluble fiber	Xylanase units (XU)

BASIC ENZYME FORMULAS FOR ANY NEED

Throughout the rest of this book, I offer suggestions for enzyme supplements to improve overall health and to treat specific ailments. Because our health is tied to the proper functioning of the main systems in our body, I rely on seventeen basic formulas that can be found online or at health food stores that carry enzyme supplements. I describe each formula in detail (what enzymes should be included and how much) each time I recommend it to make it easy to reference the information you need in one place. Following is a list of the formulas, including the key purpose of each.

- Anti-inflammatory formula: Helps address inflammation, speed recovery, and repair tissue
- Digestive formula: Helps enhance the digestion and assimilation of food while reducing the body's need to produce digestive enzymes. It is of average potency and is delivered in smaller capsules than the high potency digestive formula because of this.
- High potency digestive formula: Helps radically enhance the digestion and assimilation of food while reducing the body's need to produce digestive enzymes; the higher potency formula contains additional enzymes and averages about three times the potency of the basic digestive formula. An average formula may be substituted if three times the regular dose is taken.
- Soothing digestive formula: Helps alleviate conditions associated with gastrointestinal distress and inflammation
- High amylase formula: Helps overcome symptoms of allergies and properly digest carbohydrates, especially grains, raw vegetables, and legumes
- High cellulase formula: Helps manage yeast overgrowth
- High lipase formula: Helps improve fat digestion and metabolism, as well as the health of the cardiovascular system
- High protease formula: Helps support immune function and assist in removing viruses, fungal forms, toxins, bacteria, and heavy metals
- Nattokinase formula: Helps support cardiovascular health, decrease blood pressure and reduce the risk of inappropriate blood clots (thrombosis) by breaking down fibrin, a protein in the blood
- Nutrient enhance formula: Helps the body benefit from supplemental vitamins, minerals, and herbs
- pH balancing formula: Helps the body achieve an optimal pH (acid/alkaline) levels
- Probiotic formula: Assists the body in balancing microflora
- Mucolase formula: Helps reduce excess mucus produced by the body; particularly helpful in treating sinus and chest congestion
- Serratiopeptidase formula: Helps break down protein and reduce inflammation; supports cardiovascular health and enhances other proteases

- Antioxidant formula: Helps reduce oxidative stress
- DPPIV formula: Helps digest gluten
- Dairy digesting formula: Helps break down the common allergens in dairy

DO YOU HAVE AN ENZYME DEFICIENCY?

One of the first steps in using enzymes therapeutically should be determining if you have an enzyme deficiency. If you have one or a variety of health issues, particularly digestive problems that have been problematic for some time, it's very likely that you have an enzyme deficiency. Take the following test to help determine if and in what way you may be enzyme deficient.

ENZYME DEFICIENCY TEST

This questionnaire is intended to help you come up with a profile of your past and present nutritional habits. The information provided to help you analyze your answers is not intended to diagnose, treat, cure, or prevent any disease.

1. Which of the following best describes your body, especially when you gain weight?

    A) Gain weight evenly

    L) Carry weight in hips and thighs

    P) Carry weight in upper body, especially the stomach

    C) Has remained similar since teenage years (slim and trim, or heavy)

2. In which category is your favorite food?

    A) Carbohydrates (vegetables, breads, fruit, sweets)

    L) Rich foods, fatty foods, spicy foods

    P) Proteins (meat)

    C) Dairy

3. Which foods give you problems? Skip to the next question if specific foods do not bother you.

    A) Carbohydrates (vegetables, breads, fruit, sweets)

    L) Rich foods, fatty foods, spicy foods

    P) Proteins (meat)

    C) Dairy

4. Identify any health or physical issues you have had (present or past) in the lists below.

A) Allergies / Cold hands and feet / Depression / Fatigue / Headaches / Hemorrhoids / Low blood pressure / Neck and shoulder aches / Pancreatitis / Sprue (wheat intolerance) / Sugar cravings / Upset stomach / Ulcer

L) Aching feet / Arthritis / Bladder infections / Breast lumps / Breast tumors / Bypass surgery / Cardiovascular problems / Cataracts / Cirrhosis / Cystitis / Eczema / Fatty liver / Gallbladder problems / Gallstones / Hay fever / Hepatitis / High cholesterol / Hives / Jaundice / Prostate problems / PMS / Psoriasis / Urinary problems

P) Arteriosclerosis / Back problems / Candidiasis / Constipation / Frequent colds and flu / Ear infections / Hearing problems / Heart disease / Herniated disc / High blood pressure / Insomnia / Kidney disease / Lower back ache / Osteoporosis / Poor circulation / Sciatica

C) Chronic allergies / Colitis / Crohn's disease / Diarrhea or constipation / Diverticulosis or diverticulitis/ Irritable bowel / Milk intolerance

ANSWERS
Which letter in each question applied to you?

Question 1_____ Question 2_____ Question 3_____

In question 4, under which letter did you identify the most issues?

Question 4_____

DEFICIENCY TYPE

- Two of any letter and one of another letter suggests you have both a dominant enzyme deficiency and a secondary enzyme deficiency (most common). Your secondary deficiency is the one in the section with the lowest number.
- Two pairs of letters suggest you have two enzyme deficiencies.
- Three or four of any one letter suggests you have a dominant enzyme deficiency.
- A different letter in each section suggests you have a combination deficiency (least common).

KEY

- Type A indicates an amylase or carbohydrase deficiency (most common)
- Type L indicates a lipase deficiency
- Type P indicates a protease deficiency
- Type C indicates an amylase, lipase, and protease deficiency (combination deficiency). Please note: You cannot be both a type C and another type.

Following are diet, exercise, and enzyme therapy recommendations for each type of enzyme deficiency identified in the test. These recommendations are for primary deficiencies. If you have a primary and a secondary deficiency, consider the information provided for the secondary deficiency as an addition to the primary program where it does not conflict. You should consult a qualified medical professional before making dramatic changes to your diet or exercise regimen.

TYPE A: AMYLASE DEFICIENT

- Diet: Amylase is the enzyme that breaks down carbohydrates. Therefore, people who are amylase deficient should reduce their intake of simple carbohydrates (cakes, pies, breads, pastas), and increase their lean protein intake (if vegetarian, eat high-protein plants such as soy, beans, and nuts).

- Exercise: People who are amylase deficient need to help their bodies process and burn carbohydrates. Low impact aerobics, especially walking, three times a week, is one of the best ways to do this.

- Enzymes: A high potency digestive supplement or high amylase blend should be taken with meals. A high amylase supplement between meals can help address systemic problems associated with amylase deficiency.

TYPE L: LIPASE DEFICIENT

- Diet: Lipase is the enzyme that breaks down fats. People who are lipase deficient should reduce their intake of fatty and deep-fried foods, increase their intake of complex carbohydrates (vegetables) and lean proteins, and supplement their diet with flax oil, fish oil, or both.

- Exercise: High-energy cardiovascular exercises (depending on age) three times a week, including speed walking and jogging, are excellent types of exercise for those who are lipase deficient. This will help them burn fat that isn't being processed by the body.

- Enzymes: People who are lipase deficient should take a high potency digestive blend with meals, which should contain no less than 2,500 FCCFIP of lipase. For health issues related to lipase deficiency, a high lipase supplement three times a day on an empty stomach (no less than 5,000 FCCFIP) is helpful, particularly with flax or fish oils.

TYPE P: PROTEASE DEFICIENT

- Diet: Protease is the enzyme that breaks down proteins. People who are protease deficient should reduce their protein intake, increase their complex carbohydrate intake, and when eating protein, eat small, lean portions.

- Exercise: Cross training (resistance and cardiovascular) at least three times a week for a minimum of thirty minutes each session is one of the best exercise regimens for type P.

- Enzymes: A high potency digestive supplement with meals (no less than 70,000 HUT) and a high potency protease supplement with high protein meals and between meals for maintenance is the best enzyme therapy for people who are protease deficient.

TYPE C: COMBINATION DEFICIENT

- Diet: A combination deficiency is a deficiency in the enzymes that break down carbohydrates, fats, and proteins. Moderation and balance when eating carbohydrates, fats, and proteins are important. Protein is best consumed in the morning, and rotating food groups is beneficial. Do not eat all of the same foods all of the time. (I recommend reading *Spiritual Nutrition and the Rainbow Diet* by Gabriel Cousens if you are combination deficient.) This means not focusing too much or too long on a single food group, such as carbohydrates. It is best to have a well-balanced and varied approach to food.

- Exercise: Low-impact aerobic exercise and resistance training three times a week is a good program for type C. Tai chi would be a good choice.

- Enzymes: Type Cs should take a high potency digestive blend with meals and snacks and a high protease supplement between meals for maintenance, adding a high amylase formula and high lipase formula when the diet is shifted toward high carbohydrate or high fat meals.

FIVE SIMPLE PROGRAMS
FOR ALMOST ANYBODY

The following five enzyme therapy programs address the common needs of many people. They include immune, nutrient, and energy support, with the additions of a cleansing program and a rebuilding program. Not mentioned in each recommendation, but not to be overlooked, are the needs for a good multivitamin or greens product, essential fats (flax oil or fish oil), and plenty of purified water daily.

The enzyme formulas I recommend you use as part of these programs are not specific to a particular product or manufacturer. Rather they suggest a basic formula to look for when you are buying enzymes or enzyme blends and guidelines for using them. I refer to the same formulas repeatedly throughout this chapter and in part two of the book, but I describe them each time to make it easier for you to quickly find the information you need.

Though it may seem redundant, I recommend a digestive enzyme blend with meals as part of every program. ("With meals" means with the first bite of food you take.) Good digestion is absolutely essential to ensure optimal support when taking enzymes therapeutically.

Note that the recommendations for enzyme supplements do not provide specific amounts to be taken, just a general program for types of supplements to be taken digestively and therapeutically and approximately what those supplements should contain in terms of active units of enzymes. It is best to follow the recommendations on the supplements for amounts to be taken, adjusting them as necessary to suit your needs. Also note that the recommendations I've provided are for adults. You should consult the dosage information on the supplements to determine what is safe for children or infants.

As a general rule, however, it is good to know that there is no known threshold (maximum amount the body can utilize) for plant-based enzymes (this cannot be said for animal-sourced enzymes). This means the body will utilize and benefit from all of the enzymes consumed. This property is unique; vitamins and minerals, for example, can be overconsumed and at the point a person exceeds his threshold, they actually become a toxin to the body and can have many adverse effects. As a result plant-based enzymes are considered to be among the safest supplements you can buy.

Please note that the recommendations in this book are in no way intended to replace recommendations or advice from physicians or other health care providers. They are intended to support your path to optimal health. If you suspect you have a medical problem, I urge you to seek medical attention from a competent health care provider.

OPTIMAL DIGESTIVE AND IMMUNE SUPPORT

Enzyme deficiencies, unhealthy eating habits, exposure to environmental allergens, mycotoxins, and stress can all deplete and limit our body's capacity to digest, absorb, and assimilate foods completely. This, in turn, can compromise our immune systems. People who suffer from digestive distress such as gas, bloating, indigestion, or heartburn more than two times a week or who find themselves frequently sick will benefit from this program. To strengthen and optimize the digestive process and balance the immune system, the following products should be essential to your daily regimen.

High Potency Digestive Formula with every cooked meal

Purpose: To radically enhance the digestion and assimilation of food while reducing the body's need to produce digestive enzymes; the higher potency formula will average about three times the potency of the average digestive formula; an average formula may be substituted if three times the regular dose is taken

Each serving should contain approximately:

Amylase blend	22,000 DU	Alpha-galactosidase	450 GALU
Protease blend	80,000 HUT	Phytase	50 PU
Lipase blend	3,000 FCCFIP	Pectinase	50 AJDU
Cellulase blend	2,000 CU	Xylanase	500 XU
Invertase	80 IAU	Hemicellulase	30 HCU
Lactase	900 LacU	Beta-glucanase	25 BGU
Maltase	200 DP	L. acidophilus	250 million CFU
Glucoamylase	50 AGU		

High Protease Formula three times daily between meals

Purpose: To help support immune function and assist in removing viruses, fungal forms, toxins, bacteria, and heavy metals
Each capsule should contain approximately:

Protease blend	150,000 HUT	Serratiopeptidase	25,000 units
Mucolase	8 mg	Nattokinase blend	400 FU
Catalase	50 baker units		

pH Balancing Formula three times daily between meals

Purpose: To help the body achieve an optimal pH
Each serving should contain approximately:

Amylase blend	25,000 DU	Lipase blend	175 FCCFIP
Cellulase blend	6,000 CU	Pectinase/Phytase	200 PU
Mineral blend	Potassium bicarbonate, sodium bicarbonate, magnesium citrate	Herbal blend	Hydrilla, marshmallow, papaya
Protease blend	1,000 HUT		

The formula should not exceed 8.0 on the pH scale and the capsule should be enteric coated.

Probiotic Formula before bed

Purpose: To assist the body in balancing microflora
Each serving should contain approximately 5 billion probiotic live cells (guaranteed potency), comprised of:

Bacillus Subtillis	No less than 3 billion CFU guaranteed potency	A blend of L. acidophilus, L. casei, L. bulgaris, L. plantarum, L. rhamnosus, L. salivarius	No less than 1 billion CFU guaranteed potency
L. paracassei F-19	No less than 1 billion CFU guaranteed potency		

OPTIMAL NUTRIENT SUPPORT

Many diets and foods lack the proper quantities of vitamins and minerals that are necessary to every chemical reaction that takes place in our bodies. Deficiencies in these vital elements can lead to a host of physical imbalances and illnesses. Perhaps your hair, skin, and nails have lost their youthful look or you have frequent food cravings. If so, supplementing your diet with a pure and balanced vitamin/mineral product can supply the body with the materials that it requires to maintain and support overall health.

pH Balancing Formula at bedtime

Purpose: To help the body achieve an optimal pH
Each serving should contain approximately:

Amylase blend	25,000 DU	Lipase blend	175 FCCFIP
Cellulase blend	6,000 CU	Pectinase/Phytase	200 PU
Mineral blend	Potassium bicarbonate, sodium bicarbonate, magnesium citrate	Herbal blend	Hydrilla, marshmallow, papaya
Protease blend	1,000 HUT		

The formula should not exceed 8.0 on the pH scale and the capsule should be enteric coated.

High Protease Formula three times daily on an empty stomach

Purpose: To help support immune function and assist in removing viruses, fungal forms, toxins, bacteria, and heavy metals
Each capsule should contain approximately:

Protease blend	150,000 HUT	Serratiopeptidase	25,000 units
Mucolase	8 mg	Nattokinase blend	400 FU
Catalase	50 baker units		

High Potency Digestive Formula with every cooked meal

Purpose: To radically enhance the digestion and assimilation of food while reducing the body's need to produce digestive enzymes; the higher potency formula will average about three times the potency of the average digestive formula; an average formula may be substituted if three times the regular dose is taken

Each serving should contain approximately:

Amylase blend	22,000 DU	Alpha-galactosidase	450 GALU
Protease blend	80,000 HUT	Phytase	50 PU
Lipase blend	3,000 FCCFIP	Pectinase	50 AJDU
Cellulase blend	2,000 CU	Xylanase	500 XU
Invertase	80 IAU	Hemicellulase	30 HCU
Lactase	900 LacU	Beta-glucanase	25 BGU
Maltase	200 DP	L. acidophilus	250 million CFU
Glucoamylase	50 AGU		

Nutrient Enhance Formula with all vitamin/mineral or herb supplements consumed on empty stomach

Purpose: To help the body benefit from supplemental vitamins, minerals, and herbs
    Each serving should contain approximately:

Bioperine	5 mg	Lactase	150 ALU
Amylase blend	6,000 DU	Beta-glucanase	90 BGU
Protease blend	10,000 HUT	Xylanase	150 XU
Maltase	100 DP	Pectinase	40 PU
Glucoamylase	25 AGU	Hemicellulase	800 HCU
Alpha-galactosidase	250 GALU	Invertase	79 INVU
Lipase blend	400 FCCFIP	L. acidophilus	150 million CFU
Cellulase blend	500 CU		

OPTIMAL ENERGY AND ENDOCRINE SUPPORT

Individuals with hormonal imbalances such as chronic fatigue syndrome and fibromyalgia need extra support to maintain optimum levels of health. Optimizing the endocrine levels in the body can have the benefits of improving memory and concentration, rejuvenating the immune system, increasing overall energy, and feeding and fortifying the hypothalamus. This may also prove beneficial for individuals experiencing fatigue who have not been diagnosed with the above issues.

High Potency Digestive Formula with every cooked meal

Purpose: To radically enhance the digestion and assimilation of food while reducing the body's need to produce digestive enzymes; the higher potency formula will average about three times the potency of the average digestive formula; an average formula may be substituted if three times the regular dose is taken

Each serving should contain approximately:

Amylase blend	22,000 DU	Alpha-galactosidase	450 GALU
Protease blend	80,000 HUT	Phytase	50 PU
Lipase blend	3,000 FCCFIP	Pectinase	50 AJDU
Cellulase blend	2,000 CU	Xylanase	500 XU
Invertase	80 IAU	Hemicellulase	30 HCU
Lactase	900 LacU	Beta-glucanase	25 BGU
Maltase	200 DP	L. acidophilus	250 million CFU
Glucoamylase	50 AGU		

High Protease Formula three times daily on an empty stomach

Purpose: To help support immune function and assist in removing viruses, fungal forms, toxins, bacteria, and heavy metals

Each capsule should contain approximately:

Protease blend	150,000 HUT	Serratiopeptidase	25,000 units
Mucolase	8 mg	Nattokinase blend	400 FU
Catalase	50 baker units		

Anti-inflammatory Formula three times daily on an empty stomach

Purpose: To address inflammation, speed recovery, and repair tissue; best if enteric coated

Each serving should contain approximately:

Protease blend	120,000 HUT	Amylase blend	7,000 DU
Papain	140,000 PU	Lipase blend	600 FCCFIP
Bromelain	1,200 GDU (11.25 million FCCPU)	Catalase	100 baker units

pH Balancing Formula at bedtime

Purpose: To help the body achieve an optimal pH
Each serving should contain approximately:

Amylase blend	25,000 DU	Lipase blend	175 FCCFIP
Cellulase blend	6,000 CU	Pectinase/Phytase	200 PU
Mineral blend	Potassium bicarbonate, sodium bicarbonate, magnesium citrate	Herbal blend	Hydrilla, marshmallow, papaya
Protease blend	1,000 HUT		

The formula should not exceed 8.0 on the pH scale and the capsule should be enteric coated.

CLEANSE AND FORTIFY PROGRAM

Individuals who have very toxic bodies from years of poor food choices, heavy antibiotic use, or exposure to heavy environmental pollution, or who suspect heavy metal toxicity need to cleanse their entire digestive systems and recolonize them with healthy bacteria. Toxins, certain drugs, fungus, and chemicals in the body can interfere with the body's abilities to properly digest, absorb, and assimilate nutrients that are essential to sustaining life and health. Vital organisms that live in the digestive tract are frequently destroyed by these toxins, which in turn can ultimately deplete the immune system. Toxicity of the bowel can lead to an assault on the immune system. The toxins have been shown to penetrate the bowel lining and enter the blood. This sets off a chain reaction to which the immune system must respond. Its response often leads to an overwhelmed system that becomes underefficient, and can place an added burden on the kidneys, lungs, liver, and skin. In addition to cleansing, steps to fortify the system must also be taken to secure a healthy body and viable immune system.

High Potency Digestive Formula with every meal

Purpose: To radically enhance the digestion and assimilation of food while reducing the body's need to produce digestive enzymes; the higher potency formula will average about three times the potency of the average digestive formula; an average formula may be substituted if three times the regular dose is taken

Each serving should contain approximately:

Amylase blend	22,000 DU	Alpha-galactosidase	450 GALU
Protease blend	80,000 HUT	Phytase	50 PU
Lipase blend	3,000 FCCFIP	Pectinase	50 AJDU
Cellulase blend	2,000 CU	Xylanase	500 XU
Invertase	80 IAU	Hemicellulase	30 HCU
Lactase	900 LacU	Beta-glucanase	25 BGU
Maltase	200 DP	L. acidophilus	250 million CFU
Glucoamylase	50 AGU		

High Protease Formula three times daily on an empty stomach

Purpose: To help support immune function and assist in removing viruses, fungal forms, toxins, bacteria, and heavy metals

Each capsule should contain approximately:

Protease blend	150,000 HUT	Serratiopeptidase	25,000 units
Mucolase	8 mg	Nattokinase blend	400 FU
Catalase	50 baker units		

pH Balancing Formula three times daily

Purpose: To help the body achieve an optimal pH

Each serving should contain approximately:

Amylase blend	25,000 DU	Lipase blend	175 FCCFIP
Cellulase blend	6,000 CU	Pectinase/Phytase	200 PU
Mineral blend	Potassium bicarbonate, sodium bicarbonate, magnesium citrate	Herbal blend	Hydrilla, marshmallow, papaya
Protease blend	1,000 HUT		

The formula should not exceed 8.0 on the pH scale and the capsule should be enteric coated.

High Cellulase Formula three times a day for one week, followed by a one-month regimen of a probiotic formula at bedtime

Purpose: To manage yeast overgrowth
    Each capsule should contain approximately:

Cellulase blend	30,000 CU
Protease blend	100,000 HUT

Contraindications: High amounts of cellulase should not be taken with certain timed-release medications that contain cellulose.

Probiotic Formula before bed

Purpose: To assist the body in balancing microflora
    Each serving should contain approximately 5 billion probiotic live cells (guaranteed potency), comprised of:

Bacillus Subtillis	No less than 3 billion CFU guaranteed potency	A blend of *L. acidophilus, L. casei, L. bulgaris, L. plantarum, L. rhamnosus, L. salivarius*	No less than 1 billion CFU guaranteed potency
L. paracassei F-19	No less than 1 billion CFU guaranteed potency		

You could also add a therapeutic enzyme for a specific problem. For example, for high histamine levels, use a high amylase formula; for blood clots, use a nattokinase formula; for mucus in lungs, use a mucolase formula. See part two for specific therapies for various health problems.

REBUILD PROGRAM

The Rebuild Program is designed to aid in the overall function and maintenance of the digestive system, help restore the immune system, and provide the energy, support, and stamina needed to promote the healing and restoration necessary for obtaining restful sleep. This program is designed for the individual whose system has been compromised by stress, disease, trauma, or injury.

High Potency Digestive Formula with every meal

Purpose: To radically enhance the digestion and assimilation of food while reducing the body's need to produce digestive enzymes; the higher potency formula will average about three times the potency of the average digestive formula; an average formula may be substituted if three times the regular dose is taken

Each serving should contain approximately:

Amylase blend	22,000 DU	Alpha-galactosidase	450 GALU
Protease blend	80,000 HUT	Phytase	50 PU
Lipase blend	3,000 FCCFIP	Pectinase	50 AJDU
Cellulase blend	2,000 CU	Xylanase	500 XU
Invertase	80 IAU	Hemicellulase	30 HCU
Lactase	900 LacU	Beta-glucanase	25 BGU
Maltase	200 DP	*L. acidophilus*	250 million CFU
Glucoamylase	50 AGU		

Soothing Digestive Formula as needed

Purpose: To help alleviate conditions associated with gastrointestinal distress

Each serving should contain approximately:

Amylase blend	2,000 DU	Gotu kola	50 mg
Lipase blend	175 FCCFIP	Papaya leaf	100 mg
Cellulase blend	400 CU	Prickly ash bark	50 mg
Marshmallow root	100 mg		

Additional helpful ingredients:

DGL (deglycyrrhizinated licorice)	

This formula should *not* contain protease. Other herbs may also be present.

Serratiopeptidase Formula three times daily on an empty stomach

Purpose: To break down protein and reduce inflammation. Also supports cardiovascular health and enhances other proteases.
Each serving should contain approximately:

Serratiopeptidase	80,000 SU
Protease blend	70,000 HUT
Mineral blend	50 mg

Supporting enzymes:

Bromelain	Papain

High Protease Formula two times daily on an empty stomach, best if taken right before bed and upon rising

Purpose: To help support immune function and assist in removing viruses, fungal forms, toxins, bacteria, and heavy metals
Each capsule should contain approximately:

Protease blend	150,000 HUT	Serratiopeptidase	25,000 units
Mucolase	8 mg	Nattokinase blend	400 FU
Catalase	50 baker units		

High Amylase Formula as needed (to increase glucose levels when low energy is a symptom). Use this formula whenever you are feeling sluggish and tired. This often occurs midday.

Purpose: To overcome symptoms of allergies and for the proper digestion of carbohydrates, especially grains, raw vegetables, and legumes
Each serving should contain approximately:

Amylase blend	22,000 DU	Cellulase blend	400 CU
Glucoamylase	30 AGU	Lactase	300 LacU
Alpha-galactosidase	1,000 GALU	Maltase	300 DP
Protease blend	15,000 HUT	Pectinase	20 endo-PG
Lipase blend	150 FCCFIP		

CHOOSING THE RIGHT ENZYME SUPPLEMENT

When it's time to go to the health food store and buy an enzyme product, choosing can be a bit confusing. Often you will find that enzymes are grouped together in a way that makes little sense. The bromelain and papain products are mixed in with the digestive aids and animal-sourced enzymes (pancreatin, trypsin, and chymotrypsin). You may find detoxifying products and system cleanses on the same shelf. Often stores place these types of products with enzymes since many detoxifiers and cleanse products are directed toward the digestive system.

The key in choosing the appropriate enzyme supplement for you is to know what you are looking for. Each enzyme, whether from a plant source or an animal source, serves a unique purpose. For instance, if you are looking for an enzyme formula that can help with inflammation, then you will be looking for either a bromelain-papain blend (sold in combination or as individual ingredients; I recommend the products that combine both enzymes), or an animal-sourced enzyme blend. If you are trying to reduce stress digestively, you will be looking for a high potency plant-based (fungal, microbial) enzyme product. Once you have made this distinction, based on the information in this chapter and in part two, there are a few things to look for when picking a reputable brand.

1. Look for a company that specializes in enzymes. Often the best place to get your brakes fixed is at a shop that specializes in brakes. This is also true of tires, transmissions, paint, and so on. Companies that specialize deal exclusively in what they have become experts in. Most often you will find the best products come from companies who are not trying to be all things to all people. I suggest you buy flax oil, herbs, detoxifiers, vitamins, and teas from companies that specialize in those products. Though there are not a lot of companies that specialize in enzymes, the ones that do make very reputable and effective products. I recommend my company, Enzymedica.

2. Check the potency in the Supplement Facts. Although potency is often difficult to assess (see appendix A), the best products contain high

active units (not milligrams) with multiple strains in each category. This is often expressed as a blend of protease, lipase, or amylase. This blending will allow the enzymes to break down more protein, fat, and carbohydrates over a longer period of time.

3. Find a product with no fillers added. Many products are formulated in a way that requires fillers to be added to either fill out the capsule or help bind the tablet together. These fillers may include magnesium stearate, cellulose, pectins, talc, or similar ingredients. The fillers differ but the result is the same: a product that is less potent per milligram and runs a greater risk of containing an allergen.

4. Find a company that tests the product to ensure that it meets the label claim. Often products are blended to meet the potency printed on the label, yet by the time they have been made into capsules or tablets, some of the virtue has been lost. Reputable companies will test the finished product to make sure that what the label describes is actually in the bottle.

5. Buy enzymes in capsules (preferably vegetarian capsules) instead of tablets. Tableting is a harsh process for enzyme products, since they are more susceptible to heat and friction than ordinary vitamins. In addition, the process of tableting may also require binders or fillers.

6. Sometimes enteric-coated capsules may prove beneficial. The enteric coating serves as a barrier that prevents the enzymes from becoming active in the stomach. Instead they will be released in the small intestine, where they will be more beneficial. This may prove helpful if you are taking very large quantities of protease, if you are sensitive to supplements, or if you are experiencing extreme upper gastrointestinal inflammation.

WHERE TO PURCHASE ENZYMES

There are very few companies that specialize in enzyme supplements. A few that make good products are Enzymedica, Theramedix, Enzymatic Therapy, Renew Life, Garden of Life, Rainbow Light, Jarrow, and Transformation Enzymes. Of these, only two meet all of the above requirements. The first is Enzymedica, my company, which exclusively manufactures enzyme supplements.

These are found in most health food stores. The second company is Theramedix, which sells its products exclusively through health professionals in alternative-care facilities. Though Enzymedica and Theramedix are highly recommended, the other choices are also satisfactory. Following is the contact information for these companies.

CONSUMER PRODUCTS:

Enzymedica (carries a full line of enzyme products)
888-918-1118
www.enzymedica.com

Enzymatic Therapy (digestive and anti-inflammatory enzyme products)
800-783-2286
www.enzy.com

Renew Life (digestive and *Candida* enzyme products)
800-430-4778
www.renewlife.com

Garden of Life (digestive and anti-inflammatory enzyme products)
561-748-2477
www.gardenoflife.com

Rainbow Light
www.rainbowlight.com
800-635-1233

Jarrow
www.jarrow.com
310-204-6936

HEALTH PROFESSIONAL PRODUCTS:

Theramedix
866-998-4372
www.theramedix.net

Transformation Enzymes
713-266-2117
www.transformationenzymes.com

I hope you've found the information in this chapter and in all of part one interesting, educational, and useful. Incorporating enzyme therapy into your life is easy to do, and the benefits can be astounding. Today we are often focused on resolving symptoms of poor health, not correcting the underlying issues and improving our health for the long term. But that is the surest way to longevity; to feeling strong, healthy, and vibrant; to looking good; and to leading a full and active life.

PART TWO:
ENZYME TREATMENTS
FOR SPECIFIC
HEALTH ISSUES
(SUPPLEMENTAL ENZYME THERAPY)

HOW TO USE
THIS SECTION

In this section, various protocols are outlined to address specific ailments. There are many books on the market that outline numerous nutritional supplements for every imaginable health issue. Here I've covered the most common health problems or crises people face, and how to specifically treat them with enzyme therapy. I've based my treatment recommendations on ten years of practical application with thousands of individuals who have tested them for their effectiveness. I have not included recommendations on vitamins, herbs, and the like, though they would often prove very beneficial, since that information is readily available elsewhere.

As I mentioned in chapter 4, the enzyme formulas I recommend you use for treatment are not specific to a particular product or manufacturer. Rather I suggest a basic formula to look for when you are buying enzymes or enzyme blends and guidelines for using them. You should be able to find these formulas to purchase directly; you should not have to purchase individual enzymes or enzyme blends to create the formulas described here. In addition to the ingredients I've described for each formula, look for products that are tested by a third party, contain no fillers, and are enteric coated when necessary (see my recommendations for choosing enzyme supplements in chapter 4).

Though it may seem redundant, I recommend a digestive enzyme blend with meals for every health issue. ("With meals" means with the first bite of food you take.) Good digestion is absolutely essential to ensure optimal support when taking enzymes therapeutically, as I discussed in chapter 2.

Note that the recommendations for enzyme supplements do not provide specific amounts to be taken, just a general program for types of supplements to be taken digestively and therapeutically and approximately what those supplements should contain in terms of active units of enzymes. It is best to follow the recommendations on the supplements for amounts to be taken, adjusting them as necessary to suit your needs. Also note that the recommendations I've provided are for adults. You should consult the dosage information on the supplements to determine what is safe for children. Please note I have included a complete list of enzyme formulas that will help. The result is often a list of four or more product formulas. Because of this I have marked the most important formulas, the formulas you should not do without, with *. Please note that the recommendations in this book are in no way intended to replace recommendations or advice from physicians or other health care providers. They are intended to support your path to optimal health. If you suspect you have a medical problem, I urge you to seek medical attention from a competent health care provider.

ACNE

Acne is a chronic skin disorder caused by a variety of contributing factors. These may include, but are not limited to, hormonal imbalances, stress, inflammation of the hair follicles and the sebaceous glands, a vitamin and/or mineral deficiency, a reaction to antibiotics, candidiasis, or an inability to break down sugar and trans-fatty acids. You can improve this condition by improving your body's ability to eliminate toxins, using enzymes to improve digestion, cleanse the blood, fortify the endocrine system, and improve the assimilation of sugars and fats.

ENZYME SUPPLEMENTATION SUGGESTIONS:

*High Potency Digestive Formula with every cooked meal

Purpose: To radically enhance the digestion and assimilation of food while reducing the body's need to produce digestive enzymes; the higher potency formula will average about three times the potency of the average digestive formula; an average formula may be substituted if three times the regular dose is taken
Each serving should contain approximately:

Amylase blend	22,000 DU	Alpha-galactosidase	450 GALU
Protease blend	80,000 HUT	Phytase	50 PU
Lipase blend	3,000 FCCFIP	Pectinase	50 AJDU
Cellulase blend	2,000 CU	Xylanase	500 XU
Invertase	80 IAU	Hemicellulase	30 HCU
Lactase	900 LacU	Beta-glucanase	25 BGU
Maltase	200 DP	L. acidophilus	250 million CFU
Glucoamylase	50 AGU		

*High Protease Formula between meals

Purpose: To help support immune function and assist in removing viruses, fungal forms, toxins, bacteria, and heavy metals
Each capsule should contain approximately:

Protease blend	150,000 HUT	Serratiopeptidase	25,000 units
Mucolase	8 mg	Nattokinase blend	400 FU
Catalase	50 baker units		

ADRENAL INSUFFICIENCY

The adrenal (suprarenal) glands are the primary organ system for handling the negative effects of stress. Symptoms of adrenal insufficiency include fatigue, muscular weakness, muscle and joint pain, gastrointestinal problems, allergic hypersensitivities, hypo- or hypertension, low blood sugar, and food cravings. Adrenal insufficiency may be caused by inadequate hormone production and is often associated with poor digestion and interruptions in the production or delivery of cholesterol to the adrenal gland. You can improve this condition by using enzymes to aid digestion, balance pH levels to regulate acid production, and increase amino acid availability to support overall adrenal health.

ENZYME SUPPLEMENTATION SUGGESTIONS:

*High Potency Digestive Formula with every cooked meal

Purpose: To radically enhance the digestion and assimilation of food while reducing the body's need to produce digestive enzymes; the higher potency formula will average about three times the potency of the average digestive formula; an average formula may be substituted if three times the regular dose is taken
Each serving should contain approximately:

Amylase blend	22,000 DU	Alpha-galactosidase	450 GALU
Protease blend	80,000 HUT	Phytase	50 PU
Lipase blend	3,000 FCCFIP	Pectinase	50 AJDU
Cellulase blend	2,000 CU	Xylanase	500 XU
Invertase	80 IAU	Hemicellulase	30 HCU
Lactase	900 LacU	Beta-glucanase	25 BGU
Maltase	200 DP	L. acidophilus	250 million CFU
Glucoamylase	50 AGU		

*High Protease Formula three times daily between meals

Purpose: To help support immune function and assist in removing viruses, fungal forms, toxins, bacteria, and heavy metals
Each capsule should contain approximately:

Protease blend	150,000 HUT	Serratiopeptidase	25,000 units
Mucolase	8 mg	Nattokinase blend	400 FU
Catalase	50 baker units		

*pH Balancing Formula before bed

Purpose: To help the body achieve an optimal pH
  Each serving should contain approximately:

Amylase blend	25,000 DU	Lipase blend	175 FCCFIP
Cellulase blend	6,000 CU	Pectinase/Phytase	200 PU
Mineral blend	Potassium bicarbonate, sodium bicarbonate, magnesium citrate	Herbal blend	Hydrilla, marshmallow, papaya
Protease blend	1,000 HUT		

The formula should not exceed 8.0 on the pH scale and the capsule should be enteric coated.

AGE SPOTS

Age spots are often called liver spots. Most often seen as brown, flat spots on the skin, they are especially found on the hands, arms, and face, although as we get older, they can found almost anywhere on the body. Once thought to be harmless, they are now seen as a sign of free radical damage within the body. The spots tend to fade or disappear, however, when the liver and blood are cleansed or when the body's ability to remove free radicals is improved through improved immune function and enzyme production. Causes of this condition include excessive sun exposure, compromised liver function, the ingestion of rancid oils, a relatively poor diet, and lack of exercise.

Recommendations include liver detoxification, the addition of enzymes to a well-balanced diet, and supplemental nutritional products to improve one's overall digestion and absorption of nutrients. In addition, avoiding excess exposure to the sun and nutritional support of the hormonal and immune systems would be beneficial.

ENZYME SUPPLEMENTATION SUGGESTIONS:

*High Potency Digestive Formula with every cooked meal

Purpose: To radically enhance the digestion and assimilation of food while reducing the body's need to produce digestive enzymes; the higher potency formula will average about three times the potency of the average digestive formula; an average formula may be substituted if three times the regular dose is taken

Each serving should contain approximately:

Amylase blend	22,000 DU	Alpha-galactosidase	450 GALU
Protease blend	80,000 HUT	Phytase	50 PU
Lipase blend	3,000 FCCFIP	Pectinase	50 AJDU
Cellulase blend	2,000 CU	Xylanase	500 XU
Invertase	80 IAU	Hemicellulase	30 HCU
Lactase	900 LacU	Beta-glucanase	25 BGU
Maltase	200 DP	L. acidophilus	250 million CFU
Glucoamylase	50 AGU		

*High Protease Formula three times daily between meals

Purpose: To help support immune function and assist in removing viruses, fungal forms, toxins, bacteria, and heavy metals

Each capsule should contain approximately:

Protease blend	150,000 HUT	Serratiopeptidase	25,000 units
Mucolase	8 mg	Nattokinase blend	400 FU
Catalase	50 baker units		

High Lipase Formula three times daily between meals

Purpose: Hormone production, to improve fat digestion and metabolism, and support the endocrine system

Each capsule should contain approximately:

Lipase blend	5,000 FCCFIP	Protease blend	20,000 HUT
Amylase blend	10,000 DU	Lactase	300 LacU

AGING

Although there are no miracle cures to halt the aging process, there are healthy steps we can take to increase our life span and slow the aging process. These steps include eating a well-balanced diet high in vitamins, minerals, antioxidants, and nutrients; regular exercise; stress management; nutritional support of the hormonal and immune systems; and the addition of enzymes and supplemental nutritional products to optimize digestion and absorption of nutrients and improve the body's ability to eliminate free radicals. I also strongly recommend managing calorie intake, fasting four times a year, and eating plenty of raw food (see the nearly ideal diet on page 31).

ENZYME SUPPLEMENTATION SUGGESTIONS:

*High Potency Digestive Formula with every meal

Purpose: To radically enhance the digestion and assimilation of food while reducing the body's need to produce digestive enzymes; the higher potency formula will average about three times the potency of the average digestive formula; an average formula may be substituted if three times the regular dose is taken

Each serving should contain approximately:

Amylase blend	22,000 DU	Alpha-galactosidase	450 GALU
Protease blend	80,000 HUT	Phytase	50 PU
Lipase blend	3,000 FCCFIP	Pectinase	50 AJDU
Cellulase blend	2,000 CU	Xylanase	500 XU
Invertase	80 IAU	Hemicellulase	30 HCU
Lactase	900 LacU	Beta-glucanase	25 BGU
Maltase	200 DP	L. acidophilus	250 million CFU
Glucoamylase	50 AGU		

*Antioxidant Formula

Purpose: To reduce oxidative stress

Each serving should contain approximately:

SOD (superoxide dismutase)	75 mg	Catalase	250 baker units
Protease blend	50,000 HUT	Alpha Lopoic acid	100 mg
Glutathione	60 mg		

*pH Balancing Formula three times daily between meals

Purpose: To help the body achieve an optimal pH

Each serving should contain approximately:

Amylase blend	25,000 DU	Lipase blend	175 FCCFIP
Cellulase blend	6,000 CU	Pectinase/Phytase	200 PU
Mineral blend	Potassium bicarbonate, sodium bicarbonate, magnesium citrate	Herbal blend	Hydrilla, marshmallow, papaya
Protease blend	1,000 HUT		

The formula should not exceed 8.0 on the pH scale and the capsule should be enteric coated.

High Protease Formula three times daily between meals

Purpose: To help support immune function and assist in removing viruses, fungal forms, toxins, bacteria, and heavy metals
Each capsule should contain approximately:

Protease blend	150,000 HUT	Serratiopeptidase	25,000 units
Mucolase	8 mg	Nattokinase blend	400 FU
Catalase	50 baker units		

Anti-inflammatory Formula as needed for pain or inflammation

Purpose: To address inflammation, speed recovery, and repair tissue; best if enteric coated
Each serving should contain approximately:

Protease blend	120,000 HUT	Amylase blend	7,000 DU
Papain	140,000 PU	Lipase blend	600 FCCFIP
Bromelain	1,200 GDU (11.25 million FCCPU)	Catalase	100 baker units

ALCOHOLISM (RECOVERY)

Alcoholism is one of the most critical health problems facing today's health practitioners. More than eighteen million people in the United States (5 percent of the population) are alcoholics, although this is a rough estimate due to underreporting. The physical consequences of long-term alcohol consumption include (but are not limited to) adrenal exhaustion, brain degeneration, liver degeneration, cirrhosis of the liver, hypoglycemia, metabolic damage to cells, osteoporosis, pancreatitis, and vitamin and mineral deficiencies.

Recommendations for the recovering alcoholic include liver and blood detoxification; eating a well balanced diet with the addition of enzymes, minerals, antioxidants, and supplemental nutritional products to strengthen overall digestion and absorption of nutrients (particularly B vitamins, which many alcoholics are deficient in); and adding probiotic supplements to restore the microflora of the intestines. Aside from improved digestion and nutrient absorption, enzymes can also balance the pH of the body, strengthen the immune system, reduce inflammation, and help detoxify the body.

ENZYME SUPPLEMENTATION SUGGESTIONS:

*High Potency Digestive Formula with every meal

Purpose: To radically enhance the digestion and assimilation of food while reducing the body's need to produce digestive enzymes; the higher potency formula will average about three times the potency of the average digestive formula; an average formula may be substituted if three times the regular dose is taken
  Each serving should contain approximately:

Amylase blend	22,000 DU	Alpha-galactosidase	450 GALU
Protease blend	80,000 HUT	Phytase	50 PU
Lipase blend	3,000 FCCFIP	Pectinase	50 AJDU
Cellulase blend	2,000 CU	Xylanase	500 XU
Invertase	80 IAU	Hemicellulase	30 HCU
Lactase	900 LacU	Beta-glucanase	25 BGU
Maltase	200 DP	L. acidophilus	250 million CFU
Glucoamylase	50 AGU		

*High Protease Formula three times daily between meals

Purpose: To help support immune function and assist in removing viruses, fungal forms, toxins, bacteria, and heavy metals
  Each capsule should contain approximately:

Protease blend	150,000 HUT	Serratiopeptidase	25,000 units
Mucolase	8 mg	Nattokinase blend	400 FU
Catalase	50 baker units		

*pH Balancing Formula two times per day between meals

Purpose: To help the body achieve an optimal pH
  Each serving should contain approximately:

Amylase blend	25,000 DU	Lipase blend	175 FCCFIP
Cellulase blend	6,000 CU	Pectinase/Phytase	200 PU
Mineral blend	Potassium bicarbonate, sodium bicarbonate, magnesium citrate	Herbal blend	Hydrilla, marshmallow, papaya
Protease blend	1,000 HUT		

The formula should not exceed 8.0 on the pH scale and the capsule should be enteric coated.

High Amylase Formula as needed to raise energy levels

Purpose: To overcome symptoms of allergies and for the proper digestion of carbohydrates, especially grains, raw vegetables, and legumes

Each serving should contain approximately:

Amylase blend	22,000 DU	Cellulase blend	400 CU
Glucoamylase	30 AGU	Lactase	300 LacU
Alpha-galactosidase	1,000 GALU	Maltase	300 DP
Protease blend	15,000 HUT	Pectinase	20 endo-PG
Lipase blend	150 FCCFIP		

Probiotic Formula for a minimum of nine weeks

Purpose: To assist the body in balancing microflora

Each serving should contain approximately 5 billion probiotic live cells (guaranteed potency), comprised of:

Bacillus Subtillis	No less than 3 billion CFU guaranteed potency	A blend of *L. acidophilus, L. casei, L. bulgaris, L. plantarum, L. rhamnosus, L. salivarius*	No less than 1 billion CFU guaranteed potency
L. paracassei F-19	No less than 1 billion CFU guaranteed potency		

ALLERGIES (AIRBORNE)

Airborne allergies can be caused by a wide variety of factors: pollen, pet dander, dust, and chemicals are the most common. The allergies are caused by an oversensitive immune system that perceives these allergens to be harmful, so it launches an attack against them. This immune response most often results in allergic rhinitis, which usually involves itching, swelling or puffiness (inflammation), and excess mucus production. For some people, the response may be more severe, leading to rashes, hives, and even constriction of airways (see also ASTHMA). Allergies to pollen are often called hay fever.

Also referred to as hay fever, allergic rhinitis is an allergic response of the nasal passages and airways to air or windborne pollens. This disorder shares many common features with asthma. Nearly 75 percent of the hay fever incidences in the United States are a result of ragweed pollen. Other causative factors may include feathers, animal hair, dust and pollen from flowering plants, trees and grasses, and food allergens or sensitivities. Symptoms of hay fever may include sneezing, itchy eyes, headaches, nervous irritability, and a watery discharge from the nose and eyes.

The best treatment for allergies is to avoid the offending allergen whenever possible. It is also important to clean your living and work space often (including changing bed linens and towels) to remove as much of the allergens as possible. Enzyme therapy can be used to improve digestion, support proper and balanced functioning of the immune system, support the adrenal glands, and reduce the allergic symptoms.

ENZYME SUPPLEMENTATION SUGGESTIONS:

*High Potency Digestive Formula with every meal

Purpose: To radically enhance the digestion and assimilation of food while reducing the body's need to produce digestive enzymes; the higher potency formula will average about three times the potency of the average digestive formula; an average formula may be substituted if three times the regular dose is taken

Each serving should contain approximately:

Amylase blend	22,000 DU	Alpha-galactosidase	450 GALU
Protease blend	80,000 HUT	Phytase	50 PU
Lipase blend	3,000 FCCFIP	Pectinase	50 AJDU
Cellulase blend	2,000 CU	Xylanase	500 XU
Invertase	80 IAU	Hemicellulase	30 HCU
Lactase	900 LacU	Beta-glucanase	25 BGU
Maltase	200 DP	L. acidophilus	250 million CFU
Glucoamylase	50 AGU		

*High Amylase Formula three times daily or as needed for allergic reactions

Purpose: To overcome symptoms of allergies and for the proper digestion of carbohydrates, especially grains, raw vegetables, and legumes

Each serving should contain approximately:

Amylase blend	36,000 DU	Glucoamylase	50 AGU
Invertase	500 INVU		

High Protease Formula three times daily may be added for chronic conditions between meals

Purpose: To help support immune function and assist in removing viruses, fungal forms, toxins, bacteria, and heavy metals

Each capsule should contain approximately:

Protease blend	150,000 HUT	Serratiopeptidase	25,000 units
Mucolase	8 mg	Nattokinase blend	400 FU
Catalase	50 baker units		

Mucolase Formula as needed for nasal congestion

Purpose: To reduce excess mucus produced by the body; particularly helpful in treating sinus and chest congestion

Each serving should contain approximately:

Mucolase	30 mg

Supporting enzymes:

Amylase blend	7,000 DU	Cellulase blend	200 CU
Protease blend	20,000 HUT	Xylanase	250 XU
Glucoamylase	25 AGU	Pectinase with Phytase	175 endo-PG
Beta-glucanase	30 BGU	Hemicellulase	30 HCU
Lipase blend	250 FCCFIP	Invertase	5 INVU
Alpha-galactosidase	50 GALU		

ALLERGIES (FOOD)

It is estimated that nearly 60 percent of the American population, including 5 percent of young children, suffer from food allergies. The most common food allergens are milk, eggs, fish, shellfish, wheat, peanuts, soy, and tree nuts. Symptoms of food allergies can affect every part of the body; allergic reactions can produce mildly uncomfortable symptoms or severe illnesses. The diseases and symptoms commonly associated with food allergies can include asthma, indigestion, diarrhea, fatigue, canker sores, celiac disease, irritable bowel syndrome, hyperactivity, ear infections, migraines, bed-wetting, acne, eczema, or edema.

Many experts advocate rotation diets to identify specific food allergens. Most physicians agree that the simplest and most effective approach to treating food allergies is through the avoidance of eating allergenic foods. Since food allergies can compromise the integrity of the digestive system and exhaust the immune system, the nutritional support of these two major systems is essential. In addition, soothing the mucosal linings and removing of toxins helps. Enzymes can be used to achieve these goals and also reduce mucus production and inflammation that results from allergic reactions.

ENZYME SUPPLEMENTATION SUGGESTIONS:

*High Potency Digestive Enzyme Formula with every meal

Purpose: To radically enhance the digestion and assimilation of food while reducing the body's need to produce digestive enzymes; the higher potency formula will average about three times the potency of the average digestive formula; an average formula may be substituted if three times the regular dose is taken

Each serving should contain approximately:

Amylase blend	22,000 DU	Alpha-galactosidase	450 GALU
Protease blend	80,000 HUT	Phytase	50 PU
Lipase blend	3,000 FCCFIP	Pectinase	50 AJDU
Cellulase blend	2,000 CU	Xylanase	500 XU
Invertase	80 IAU	Hemicellulase	30 HCU
Lactase	900 LacU	Beta-glucanase	25 BGU
Maltase	200 DP	L. acidophilus	250 million CFU
Glucoamylase	50 AGU		

Many of the foods people are sensitive to are carbohydrates, in which cases a high amylase formula would be recommended with meals. Other sensitivities (allergies) are reactions to one specific type of food, such as dairy, or foods that contain the protein gluten. These can be addressed with specific enzyme formulas that contain the enzymes that address these foods.

*Dairy Digesting Formula for lactose sensitivity whenever dairy is eaten

Purpose: To help break down the common allergens in dairy, which includes lactose and casein

Each serving should contain approximately:

Lactase	9,000 ALU	Amylase blend	7,500 DU
Protease blend	25,000 HUT	Glucoamylase	25 AG
Lipase blend	500 FCCFIP	Malstase	350 DP
Cellulase	300 CU		

*DPPIV Formula for wheat or gluten sensitivities whenever those foods are consumed or when eating out to prevent gluten crossover contamination

Purpose: To digest gluten (a common allergen found in wheat and cereal grains). DPPIV has proven helpful for individuals who are sensitive to gluten.

Each serving should contain approximately:

DPPIV Protease blend	80,000 HUT	Glucoamylase	15,000 AGU
Amylase blend	15,000 DU		

*Probiotic Formula daily before bed

Purpose: To assist the body in balancing microflora
Each serving should contain approximately 5 billion probiotic live cells (guaranteed potency), comprised of:

Bacillus Subtillis	No less than 3 billion CFU guaranteed potency	A blend of *L. acidophilus, L. casei, L. bulgaris, L. plantarum, L. rhamnosus, L. salivarius*	No less than 1 billion CFU guaranteed potency
L. paracassei F-19	No less than 1 billion CFU guaranteed potency		

Soothing Digestive Formula as needed for abdominal pain

Purpose: To help alleviate conditions associated with gastrointestinal distress
Each serving should contain approximately:

Amylase blend	2,000 DU	Gotu kola	50 mg
Lipase blend	175 FCCFIP	Papaya leaf	100 mg
Cellulase blend	400 CU	Prickly ash bark	50 mg
Marshmallow root	100 mg		

Additional helpful ingredients:

DGL (deglycyrrhizinated licorice)	

This formula should *not* contain protease. Other herbs may also be present.

Mucolase Formula or High Amylase Formula as needed for reactions or mucus

Purpose: To reduce excess mucus produced by the body; particularly helpful in treating sinus and chest congestion

Each serving should contain approximately:

Mucolase	30 mg

Supporting enzymes:

Amylase blend	7,000 DU	Cellulase blend	200 CU
Protease blend	20,000 HUT	Xylanase	250 XU
Glucoamylase	25 AGU	Pectinase with Phytase	175 endo-PG
Beta-glucanase	30 BGU	Hemicellulase	30 HCU
Lipase blend	250 FCCFIP	Invertase	5 INVU
Alpha-galactosidase	50 GALU		

Purpose: To overcome symptoms of allergies and for the proper digestion of carbohydrates, especially grains, raw vegetables, and legumes

Each serving should contain approximately:

Amylase blend	22,000 DU	Cellulase blend	400 CU
Glucoamylase	30 AGU	Lactase	300 LacU
Alpha-galactosidase	1,000 GALU	Maltase	300 DP
Protease blend	15,000 HUT	Pectinase	20 endo-PG
Lipase blend	150 FCCFIP		

ALZHEIMER'S DISEASE

Alzheimer's disease is a degenerative brain disorder afflicting 4.5 million Americans. It affects those parts of the brain that control thought, memory, and language. The symptoms of Alzheimer's disease are progressive mental deterioration characterized by an inability to carry out daily activities, a loss of cognitive functions, and a loss of memory functions. Extensive research studies indicate that the causes of Alzheimer's disease can include genetic factors, age, environmental factors, chronic exposure to aluminum and/or silicon, and increased oxidative damage due to long-term toxic exposure.

Recommendations include a healthy, well-balanced diet and lifestyle; avoidance of products that contain mercury and aluminum (which include antiperspirants, antacids, baking powder, and aluminum cookware); and increasing antioxidant levels in the body. Nutritional supplementation with high-potency vitamins, minerals, antioxidants, and particularly magnesium and potassium products are beneficial. Enzymes can be used to support the absorption of nutrients, improve overall health through an improved pH balance, increase the level of antioxidant enzymes in the body, and even improve nerve communication.

ENZYME SUPPLEMENTATION SUGGESTIONS:

*High Potency Digestive Formula with every meal

Purpose: To radically enhance the digestion and assimilation of food while reducing the body's need to produce digestive enzymes; the higher potency formula will average about three times the potency of the average digestive formula; an average formula may be substituted if three times the regular dose is taken

Each serving should contain approximately:

Amylase blend	22,000 DU	Alpha-galactosidase	450 GALU
Protease blend	80,000 HUT	Phytase	50 PU
Lipase blend	3,000 FCCFIP	Pectinase	50 AJDU
Cellulase blend	2,000 CU	Xylanase	500 XU
Invertase	80 IAU	Hemicellulase	30 HCU
Lactase	900 LacU	Beta-glucanase	25 BGU
Maltase	200 DP	L. acidophilus	250 million CFU
Glucoamylase	50 AGU		

*Antioxidant Formula at least two times a day on an empty stomach

Purpose: To reduce oxidative stress
Each serving should contain approximately:

SOD (superoxide dismutase)	75 mg	Catalase	250 baker units
Protease blend	50,000 HUT	Alpha Lopoic acid	100 mg
Glutathione	60 mg		

*Nattokinase Formula three times daily between meals

Purpose: To increase circulation and break down fibrin
Each serving should contain approximately:
Necessary ingredient:

Nattokinase NSK-SD	1,000 FU

Helpful ingredients:

Amylase blend	9,000 DU	Glucoamylase	25 AGU
Protease blend	20,000 HUT	Lipase blend	1,000 FCCFIP
Minerals	85 mg	Cellulase blend	400 CU

High Protease Formula three times daily on an empty stomach

Purpose: To help support immune function and assist in removing viruses, fungal forms, toxins, bacteria, and heavy metals
    Each capsule should contain approximately:

Protease blend	150,000 HUT	Serratiopeptidase	25,000 units
Mucolase	8 mg	Nattokinase blend	400 FU
Catalase	50 baker units		

pH Balancing Formula three times daily

Purpose: To help the body achieve an optimal pH
    Each serving should contain approximately:

Amylase blend	25,000 DU	Lipase blend	175 FCCFIP
Cellulase blend	6,000 CU	Pectinase/Phytase	200 PU
Mineral blend	Potassium bicarbonate, sodium bicarbonate, magnesium citrate	Herbal blend	Hydrilla, marshmallow, papaya
Protease blend	1,000 HUT		

The formula should not exceed 8.0 on the pH scale and the capsule should be enteric coated.

ANEMIA

Anemia is a blood disorder that results in a lower than normal number of red blood cells in the blood. The concentration of the oxygen-carrying pigment (hemoglobin) in the blood is below normal. Anemia can be caused by excessive blood loss, excessive red blood cell destruction, iron deficiency, and/or deficient red blood cell production. Symptoms of anemia include weakness, fatigue, pallor, headaches, heart palpitations, shortness of breath, bruising easily, nosebleeds, bleeding gums, or frequent infections.

A blood test for anemia may show a low volume of blood, a low level of total red blood cells, or red blood cells of an abnormal size or shape (i.e., sickle cell anemia). Identifying the underlying cause of anemia through a complete diagnostic evaluation is essential. When treating anemia, it is critical to support the digestive and immune systems and restore energy through improving the absorption of vital minerals and vitamins, particularly iron. Enzyme therapy supports all of these goals and can also be used to help the body maintain a correct pH balance.

ENZYME SUPPLEMENTATION SUGGESTIONS:

*High Potency Digestive Formula with every meal

Purpose: To radically enhance the digestion and assimilation of food while reducing the body's need to produce digestive enzymes; the higher potency formula will average about three times the potency of the average digestive formula; an average formula may be substituted if three times the regular dose is taken

Each serving should contain approximately:

Amylase blend	22,000 DU	Alpha-galactosidase	450 GALU
Protease blend	80,000 HUT	Phytase	50 PU
Lipase blend	3,000 FCCFIP	Pectinase	50 AJDU
Cellulase blend	2,000 CU	Xylanase	500 XU
Invertase	80 IAU	Hemicellulase	30 HCU
Lactase	900 LacU	Beta-glucanase	25 BGU
Maltase	200 DP	L. acidophilus	250 million CFU
Glucoamylase	50 AGU		

*High Protease Formula three times daily

Purpose: To help support immune function and assist in removing viruses, fungal forms, toxins, bacteria, and heavy metals
Each capsule should contain approximately:

Protease blend	150,000 HUT	Serratiopeptidase	25,000 units
Mucolase	8 mg	Nattokinase blend	400 FU
Catalase	50 baker units		

pH Balancing Formula three times daily

Purpose: To help the body achieve an optimal pH
Each serving should contain approximately:

Amylase blend	25,000 DU	Lipase blend	175 FCCFIP
Cellulase blend	6,000 CU	Pectinase/Phytase	200 PU
Mineral blend	Potassium bicarbonate, sodium bicarbonate, magnesium citrate	Herbal blend	Hydrilla, marshmallow, papaya
Protease blend	1,000 HUT		

The formula should not exceed 8.0 on the pH scale and the capsule should be enteric coated.

ANXIETY

Anxiety is an emotional state that can range in intensity from unease to intense fear. It is estimated that over four million Americans suffer from anxiety. Anxiety becomes symptomatic when it starts to inhibit thoughts and feelings and disrupt normal activities of daily life. Some of the most common symptoms include back pain, heart palpitations, excessive sweating, headaches, an inability to take in enough air, a tendency either to hyperventilate or sigh repeatedly, dizziness, digestive disturbances, and muscle tightness. Long-term anxiety is a severe stressor on the body and can deplete the body of nutrients and minerals and contribute to glandular and hormonal imbalances.

Recommendations include avoiding caffeine, sugar, food allergens, and alcohol, all of which can contribute directly to anxiety levels or reduce the ability to manage stress. Other recommended practices include eating regular healthy meals in a relaxed atmosphere; incorporating relaxation, breathing exercises, and moderate physical exercise into one's daily routine; and eliminating or reducing the sources of stress. Enzyme therapy can be used to improve digestion, improve pH balance in the body, and support the functioning of the immune system, all of which can suffer from the systemic negative effects of anxiety. In addition, people who suffer severe bouts of anxiety can use enzyme supplements to reduce sugar cravings, which often occur with stress.

ENZYME SUPPLEMENTATION SUGGESTIONS:

*High Potency Digestive Formula with every meal

Purpose: To radically enhance the digestion and assimilation of food while reducing the body's need to produce digestive enzymes; the higher potency formula will average about three times the potency of the average digestive formula; an average formula may be substituted if three times the regular dose is taken
Each serving should contain approximately:

Amylase blend	22,000 DU	Alpha-galactosidase	450 GALU
Protease blend	80,000 HUT	Phytase	50 PU
Lipase blend	3,000 FCCFIP	Pectinase	50 AJDU
Cellulase blend	2,000 CU	Xylanase	500 XU
Invertase	80 IAU	Hemicellulase	30 HCU
Lactase	900 LacU	Beta-glucanase	25 BGU
Maltase	200 DP	L. acidophilus	250 million CFU
Glucoamylase	50 AGU		

*High Protease Formula three times daily between meals

Purpose: To help support immune function and assist in removing viruses, fungal forms, toxins, bacteria, and heavy metals
  Each capsule should contain approximately:

Protease blend	150,000 HUT	Serratiopeptidase	25,000 units
Mucolase	8 mg	Nattokinase blend	400 FU
Catalase	50 baker units		

*pH Balancing Formula three times daily between meals

Purpose: To help the body achieve an optimal pH
  Each serving should contain approximately:

Amylase blend	25,000 DU	Lipase blend	175 FCCFIP
Cellulase blend	6,000 CU	Pectinase/Phytase	200 PU
Mineral blend	Potassium bicarbonate, sodium bicarbonate, magnesium citrate	Herbal blend	Hydrilla, marshmallow, papaya
Protease blend	1,000 HUT		

The formula should not exceed 8.0 on the pH scale and the capsule should be enteric coated.

High Amylase Formula when food cravings arise

Purpose: To overcome symptoms of allergies and for the proper digestion of carbohydrates, especially grains, raw vegetables, and legumes
  Each serving should contain approximately:

Amylase blend	22,000 DU	Cellulase blend	400 CU
Glucoamylase	30 AGU	Lactase	300 LacU
Alpha-galactosidase	1,000 GALU	Maltase	300 DP
Protease blend	15,000 HUT	Pectinase	20 endo-PG
Lipase blend	150 FCCFIP		

ARTHRITIS

Arthritis is characterized by inflammation, pain, swelling, stiffness, and redness of the joints. The two primary types of arthritis include osteoarthritis and rheumatoid arthritis. The symptoms can vary from slight discomfort to complete debilitation.

Osteoarthritis (degenerative arthritis) is the most common type of arthritis. It most often results from wear and tear on the joints that causes degeneration of the cartilage around the joint and eventually damage to the bone. It is prevalent in older people. A focus on improving joint health early in life through regular exercise and healthy meals to support the body's ability to repair tissues is the best way to avoid the symptoms of osteoarthritis later in life. Rheumatoid arthritis is an autoimmune disorder. It is the most severe type of inflammatory joint disease. The body's immune system acts against and damages the surrounding soft tissues (muscles, tendons, ligaments) of joints and eventually damages the joints themselves. As a result, the joints in the hands, feet, and/or arms become extremely painful, stiff, and eventually deformed.

Enzyme therapy has been used to treat arthritis for many years, particularly because of the ability of certain enzymes to reduce inflammation. Enzymes also improve circulation, support tissue repair, and improve nutrient absorption and pH balance to improve overall health of the body's tissues.

ENZYME SUPPLEMENTATION SUGGESTIONS:

*High Potency Digestive Formula with every meal

Purpose: To radically enhance the digestion and assimilation of food while reducing the body's need to produce digestive enzymes; the higher potency formula will average about three times the potency of the average digestive formula; an average formula may be substituted if three times the regular dose is taken

Each serving should contain approximately:

Amylase blend	22,000 DU	Alpha-galactosidase	450 GALU
Protease blend	80,000 HUT	Phytase	50 PU
Lipase blend	3,000 FCCFIP	Pectinase	50 AJDU
Cellulase blend	2,000 CU	Xylanase	500 XU
Invertase	80 IAU	Hemicellulase	30 HCU
Lactase	900 LacU	Beta-glucanase	25 BGU
Maltase	200 DP	L. acidophilus	250 million CFU
Glucoamylase	50 AGU		

*Anti-inflammatory Formula three times daily between meals (with an additional amount used if needed)

Purpose: To address inflammation, speed recovery, and repair tissue; best if enteric coated

Each serving should contain approximately:

Protease blend	120,000 HUT	Amylase blend	7,000 DU
Papain	140,000 PU	Lipase blend	600 FCCFIP
Bromelain	1,200 GDU (11.25 million FCCPU)	Catalase	100 baker units

Serratiopeptidase Formula may be added every time the anti-inflammatory formula is taken when there is chronic pain

Purpose: To break down protein and reduce inflammation. Also supports cardiovascular health and enhances other proteases.

Each serving should contain approximately:

Serratiopeptidase	80,000 SU
Protease blend	70,000 HUT
Mineral blend	50 mg

Supporting enzymes:

Bromelain	Papain

pH Balancing Formula three times daily between meals

Purpose: To help the body achieve an optimal pH

Each serving should contain approximately:

Amylase blend	25,000 DU	Lipase blend	175 FCCFIP
Cellulase blend	6,000 CU	Pectinase/Phytase	200 PU
Mineral blend	Potassium bicarbonate, sodium bicarbonate, magnesium citrate	Herbal blend	Hydrilla, marshmallow, papaya
Protease blend	1,000 HUT		

The formula should not exceed 8.0 on the pH scale and the capsule should be enteric coated.

Optional: High Protease Formula three times daily between meals

Purpose: To help support immune function and assist in removing viruses, fungal forms, toxins, bacteria, and heavy metals

Each capsule should contain approximately:

Protease blend	150,000 HUT	Serratiopeptidase	25,000 units
Mucolase	8 mg	Nattokinase blend	400 FU
Catalase	50 baker units		

ASTHMA

Asthma is a breathing disorder characterized by inflammation and narrowing of the airways in the trachea and lungs, particularly the bronchioles in the lungs. The symptoms of asthma are recurrent attacks of breathlessness, tightness in the chest, and wheezing when exhaling.

The two main types of asthma are extrinsic and intrinsic. Extrinsic asthma is an allergic response to something inhaled, and heredity seems to be a major factor in development. Frequently beginning in childhood, extrinsic asthma often becomes less severe as a person ages. Intrinsic asthma tends to develop later in life and often follows a respiratory tract infection. Emotional factors, such as stress or anxiety, may precipitate attacks of intrinsic asthma.

Recommendations include using enzyme therapy to provide support of the digestive and immune systems, help to heal irritated mucosal linings, and reduce inflammation. Avoiding airborne and food allergens, cleansing the system through elimination diets, and managing stress are also very beneficial.

ENZYME SUPPLEMENTATION SUGGESTIONS:

*High Potency Digestive Formula or High Amylase Formula with every meal

Purpose: To radically enhance the digestion and assimilation of food while reducing the body's need to produce digestive enzymes; the higher potency formula will average about three times the potency of the average digestive formula; an average formula may be substituted if three times the regular dose is taken

Each serving should contain approximately:

Amylase blend	22,000 DU	Alpha-galactosidase	450 GALU
Protease blend	80,000 HUT	Phytase	50 PU
Lipase blend	3,000 FCCFIP	Pectinase	50 AJDU
Cellulase blend	2,000 CU	Xylanase	500 XU
Invertase	80 IAU	Hemicellulase	30 HCU
Lactase	900 LacU	Beta-glucanase	25 BGU
Maltase	200 DP	L. acidophilus	250 million CFU
Glucoamylase	50 AGU		

*Serratiopeptidase Formula three times a day on an empty stomach

Purpose: To break down protein and reduce inflammation. Also supports cardiovascular health and enhances other proteases.

Each serving should contain approximately:

Serratiopeptidase	80,000 SU
Protease blend	70,000 HUT
Mineral blend	50 mg

Supporting enzymes:

Bromelain	Papain

High Amylase Formula three times daily

Purpose: To overcome symptoms of allergies and for the proper digestion of carbohydrates, especially grains, raw vegetables, and legumes

Each serving should contain approximately:

Amylase blend	22,000 DU	Cellulase blend	400 CU
Glucoamylase	30 AGU	Lactase	300 LacU
Alpha-galactosidase	1,000 GALU	Maltase	300 DP
Protease blend	15,000 HUT	Pectinase	20 endo-PG
Lipase blend	150 FCCFIP		

High Protease Formula three times daily between meals

Purpose: To help support immune function and assist in removing viruses, fungal forms, toxins, bacteria, and heavy metals

Each capsule should contain approximately:

Protease blend	150,000 HUT	Serratiopeptidase	25,000 units
Mucolase	8 mg	Nattokinase blend	400 FU
Catalase	50 baker units		

ATHLETE'S FOOT

See RINGWORM.

ATHLETIC PERFORMANCE

Athletes are always looking for ways to perform at peak levels, and enzymes can assist them in doing that. Proteases in particular can be beneficial, especially in helping the athlete recover after intense physical activity. For example, in a recent study, runners were given protease supplements or a placebo four times a day for three days, twenty-four hours before and forty-eight hours after running. Evaluation of the participants found less soreness, improved pain threshold, and no mood change with those taking the protease supplements over the group who took the placebo. Enhanced recovery can improve overall physical performance.

The enzyme support mechanism for athletic performance is tied to circulation and oxygen availability. Proteolytic enzymes help the blood circulate more effectively throughout the body by reducing fibrin (a protein produced in the blood that causes blood to clot), which can decrease circulation and reduce oxygen uptake. The more efficiently the blood travels through the many miles of veins and arteries, the more long-term energy an athlete has to feed the muscles the oxygen required during hard physical labor or exercise. (See also ENERGY AND ENDURANCE.) Strenuous exercise also produces acid, so keeping the body in balance may also help speed recovery.

ENZYME SUPPLEMENTATION SUGGESTIONS:

*High Potency Digestive Formula with every meal

Purpose: To radically enhance the digestion and assimilation of food while reducing the body's need to produce digestive enzymes; the higher potency formula will average about three times the potency of the average digestive formula; an average formula may be substituted if three times the regular dose is taken

Each serving should contain approximately:

Amylase blend	22,000 DU	Alpha-galactosidase	450 GALU
Protease blend	80,000 HUT	Phytase	50 PU
Lipase blend	3,000 FCCFIP	Pectinase	50 AJDU
Cellulase blend	2,000 CU	Xylanase	500 XU
Invertase	80 IAU	Hemicellulase	30 HCU
Lactase	900 LacU	Beta-glucanase	25 BGU
Maltase	200 DP	L. acidophilus	250 million CFU
Glucoamylase	50 AGU		

*Anti-inflammatory Formula before and immediately after strenuous exercise

Purpose: To address inflammation, speed recovery, and repair tissue; best if enteric coated

Each serving should contain approximately:

Protease blend	120,000 HUT	Amylase blend	7,000 DU
Papain	140,000 PU	Lipase blend	600 FCCFIP
Bromelain	1,200 GDU (11.25 million FCCPU)	Catalase	100 baker units

pH Balancing Formula after strenuous exercise and before bed

Purpose: To help the body achieve an optimal pH

Each serving should contain approximately:

Amylase blend	25,000 DU	Lipase blend	175 FCCFIP
Cellulase blend	6,000 CU	Pectinase/Phytase	200 PU
Mineral blend	Potassium bicarbonate, sodium bicarbonate, magnesium citrate	Herbal blend	Hydrilla, marshmallow, papaya
Protease blend	1,000 HUT		

The formula should not exceed 8.0 on the pH scale and the capsule should be enteric coated.

High Protease formula before bed and upon rising

Purpose: To help support immune function and assist in removing viruses, fungal forms, toxins, bacteria, and heavy metals

Each capsule should contain approximately:

Protease blend	150,000 HUT	Serratiopeptidase	25,000 units
Mucolase	8 mg	Nattokinase blend	400 FU
Catalase	50 baker units		

ATTENTION DEFICIT/HYPERACTIVITY DISORDER

Attention deficit/hyperactivity disorder (ADHD) can affect both children and adults. The symptoms may include one or more of the following: inability to concentrate, impulsiveness, hyperactivity, impatience, self-destructiveness, quick frustration, temper tantrums, sleep disturbances, clumsiness, failure in the class-room, and difficulty developing or maintaining peer relationships. There are vari-ous types and severity levels of ADHD, so it is important for children or adults with these types of behavioral issues to be evaluated by a medical expert.

The exact causes of ADHD are not known, but contributing factors include oxygen deprivation at birth, prenatal trauma, heredity, food allergies and artifi-cial additives in food (particularly foods containing salicylates), smoking during pregnancy, lead poisoning, a low-protein diet, a protease deficiency, and environ-mental pollutants.

Recommendations include diagnostic tests and evaluations to ascertain the underlying cause of the condition, eating a well-balanced diet and avoiding sugars and foods with a high glycemic index, and ruling out or treating sensitivities or allergies to foods, preservatives, additives, and/or environmental toxins. Also rec-ommended are detoxification and drainage products to regenerate the liver, lymph system, and blood cleansing process. Enzymes and nutritional products can sup-port the digestive and immune systems.

ENZYME SUPPLEMENTATION SUGGESTIONS:

*Digestive Formula with every meal and snack

Purpose: To enhance the digestion and assimilation of food while reducing the body's need to produce digestive enzymes

Each serving should contain approximately:

Necessary Ingredients:

Amylase blend	12,000 DU	Alpha-galactosidase	75 GALU
Protease blend	42,000 HUT	Lipase blend	500 FCCFIP
Invertase	10 IAU	Lactase	850 LacU
Maltase	200 DP	Phytase	50 PU
Cellulase blend	200 CU	Pectinase	50 AJDU

Helpful Ingredients:

Xylanase	L. acidophilus
Beta-glucanase	L. bifidus
Hemicellulase	

*pH Balancing Formula before bed

Purpose: To help the body achieve an optimal pH

Each serving should contain approximately:

Amylase blend	25,000 DU	Lipase blend	175 FCCFIP
Cellulase blend	6,000 CU	Pectinase/Phytase	200 PU
Mineral blend	Potassium bicarbonate, sodium bicarbonate, magnesium citrate	Herbal blend	Hydrilla, marshmallow, papaya
Protease blend	1,000 HUT		

The formula should not exceed 8.0 on the pH scale and the capsule should be enteric coated.

High Protease Formula three to four times per day (for detoxification)

Purpose: To help support immune function and assist in removing viruses, fungal forms, toxins, bacteria, and heavy metals

Each capsule should contain approximately:

Protease blend	150,000 HUT	Serratiopeptidase	25,000 units
Mucolase	8 mg	Nattokinase blend	400 FU
Catalase	50 baker units		

AUTISM

Autism is a neurobiological developmental disorder affecting 1 out of every 160 children. Autistic children demonstrate deficits in social interaction, limited development of verbal and nonverbal communication, and repetitive behaviors or interests. The symptoms of autism range from very mild to severe. Speech development is often delayed or absent. Some children exhibit nonsense babbling and may be unresponsive or resistant to signs of affection or human contact. Many of these children have learning disabilities, are withdrawn, or have unusual responses to sensory experiences. Behavior can range from total silence to periods of hyperactivity that may include self-abuse. The cause of autism is not known.

Recommendations include support of the digestive and immune systems and ruling out food allergies, chemical sensitivities, and heavy metal toxicity. For more information about using enzymes for autism, refer to *Enzymes for Autism and Other Neurological Conditions* by Karen DeFelice (Thundersnow, 2002).

ENZYME SUPPLEMENTATION SUGGESTIONS

It is best when addressing these issues with enzymes to start with a low dosage one or two times daily. People with autism tend to be more sensitive and do best when the supplemental recommendations are eased into (low and slow).

*High Amylase Formula with every meal (low and slow)

Purpose: To overcome symptoms of allergies and for the proper digestion of carbohydrates, especially grains, raw vegetables, and legumes
Each serving should contain approximately:

Amylase blend	22,000 DU	Cellulase blend	400 CU
Glucoamylase	30 AGU	Lactase	300 LacU
Alpha-galactosidase	1,000 GALU	Maltase	300 DP
Protease blend	15,000 HUT	Pectinase	20 endo-PG
Lipase blend	150 FCCFIP		

* Probiotic Formula before bed daily

Purpose: To assist the body in balancing microflora
Each serving should contain approximately 5 billion probiotic live cells (guaranteed potency), comprised of:

Bacillus Subtillis	No less than 3 billion CFU guaranteed potency	A blend of L. acidophilus, L. casei, L. bulgaris, L. plantarum, L. rhamnosus, L. salivarius	No less than 1 billion CFU guaranteed potency
L. paracassei F-19	No less than 1 billion CFU guaranteed potency		

* High Protease Formula three times daily between meals (low and slow) when immune system support is needed

Purpose: To help support immune function and assist in removing viruses, fungal forms, toxins, bacteria, and heavy metals
Each capsule should contain approximately:

Protease blend	150,000 HUT	Serratiopeptidase	25,000 units
Mucolase	8 mg	Nattokinase blend	400 FU
Catalase	50 baker units		

*DPPIV Formula whenever foods containing gluten are eaten or there is potential that foods eaten have been cooked with foods containing gluten (such as when eating out)

Purpose: To digest gluten (a common allergen found in wheat and cereal grains). DPPIV has proven helpful for individuals who are sensitive to gluten.

Each serving should contain approximately:

DPPIV Protease blend	80,000 HUT	Glucoamylase	15,000 AGU
Amylase blend	15,000 DU		

Soothing Digestive Formula as needed

Purpose: To help alleviate conditions associated with gastrointestinal distress
Each serving should contain approximately:

Amylase blend	2,000 DU	Gotu kola	50 mg
Lipase blend	175 FCCFIP	Papaya leaf	100 mg
Cellulase blend	400 CU	Prickly ash bark	50 mg
Marshmallow root	100 mg		

Additional helpful ingredients:

DGL (deglycyrrhizinated licorice)	

This formula should *not* contain protease. Other herbs may also be present.

pH Balancing Formula three times daily

Purpose: To help the body achieve an optimal pH
Each serving should contain approximately:

Amylase blend	25,000 DU	Lipase blend	175 FCCFIP
Cellulase blend	6,000 CU	Pectinase/Phytase	200 PU
Mineral blend	Potassium bicarbonate, sodium bicarbonate, magnesium citrate	Herbal blend	Hydrilla, marshmallow, papaya
Protease blend	1,000 HUT		

The formula should not exceed 8.0 on the pH scale and the capsule should be enteric coated.

Dairy Digesting Formula for lactose sensitivity whenever dairy is eaten

Purpose: To help break down the common allergens in dairy, which includes lactose and casein
Each serving should contain approximately:

Lactase	9,000 ALU	Amylase blend	7,500 DU
Protease blend	25,000 HUT	Glucoamylase	25 AG
Lipase blend	500 FCCFIP	Malstase	350 DP
Cellulase	300 CU		

BACKACHE

Backaches can involve disorders of the bones, muscles, nerves, joints, ligaments, and tendons of the spine. The most common cause of chronic back pain is injury, but other common causes can include poor posture, stress, arthritis, bone disease, scoliosis, and slipped discs. Another possible cause of back pain is kidney infection or kidney stones (See KIDNEY STRESS).

Recommendations are dependent upon a thorough evaluation of the possible causative factors, but enzymes can be used to treat inflammation and to support the body's ability to repair tissue through nutrient absorption and availability of amino acids.

ENZYME SUPPLEMENTATION SUGGESTIONS:

*Anti-inflammatory Formula three times daily (more may be used as needed)

Purpose: To address inflammation, speed recovery, and repair tissue; best if enteric coated

Each serving should contain approximately:

Protease blend	120,000 HUT	Amylase blend	7,000 DU
Papain	140,000 PU	Lipase blend	600 FCCFIP
Bromelain	1,200 GDU (11.25 million FCCPU)	Catalase	100 baker units

High Potency Digestive Formula with every meal

Purpose: To radically enhance the digestion and assimilation of food while reducing the body's need to produce digestive enzymes; the higher potency formula will average about three times the potency of the average digestive formula; an average formula may be substituted if three times the regular dose is taken

Each serving should contain approximately:

Amylase blend	22,000 DU	Alpha-galactosidase	450 GALU
Protease blend	80,000 HUT	Phytase	50 PU
Lipase blend	3,000 FCCFIP	Pectinase	50 AJDU
Cellulase blend	2,000 CU	Xylanase	500 XU
Invertase	80 IAU	Hemicellulase	30 HCU
Lactase	900 LacU	Beta-glucanase	25 BGU
Maltase	200 DP	L. acidophilus	250 million CFU
Glucoamylase	50 AGU		

Serratiopeptidase Formula may be added to the anti-inflammatory enzyme formula for chronic pain

Purpose: To break down protein and reduce inflammation. Also supports cardiovascular health and enhances other proteases.

Each serving should contain approximately:

Serratiopeptidase	80,000 SU
Protease blend	70,000 HUT
Mineral blend	50 mg

Supporting enzymes:

Bromelain	Papain

BACTERIAL VAGINOSIS

Bacterial vaginosis (BV) is a condition in which the normal balance of bacteria in the vagina is disrupted and replaced by an overgrowth of certain bacteria that are considered to be harmful to the natural state of the vagina. The most common symptoms are discharge, a strong fishy odor, pain, itching, and burning. The symptoms are easily confused with those of a yeast infection (CANDIDIASIS) and women often treat it with over-the-counter medicines for yeast infection. However, BV is far more common than yeast infection. In fact, it is the most common vaginal infection. The primary differences between the two are that BV is usually associated with a heavy discharge that has a strong fishy odor, and a yeast infection doesn't usually involve such an odor. Also, BV may involve some mild burning or itching, but with yeast infections, that symptom is more common and more intense.

Not much is known about how women get BV. However, some activities or behaviors can upset the normal balance of bacteria in the vagina, including douching, using an intrauterine device (IUD) for contraception, and having a new sexual partner or multiple sexual partners.

It is important to treat BV because it can increase a woman's risk for pelvic inflammatory disease, increase her susceptibility for contracting other diseases, and cause problems during pregnancy. Pregnant women with BV more often have babies who are born premature or with low birth weight. If you suspect you have BV, you should see your doctor.

BV is treated with antibiotic therapy. Enzyme therapy can be used to cleanse the body of the *Candida* overgrowth and deter its return.

*Digestive Formula with each meal

Purpose: To enhance the digestion and assimilation of food while reducing the body's need to produce digestive enzymes
Each serving should contain approximately:
Necessary Ingredients:

Amylase blend	12,000 DU	Alpha-galactosidase	75 GALU
Protease blend	42,000 HUT	Lipase blend	500 FCCFIP
Invertase	10 IAU	Lactase	850 LacU
Maltase	200 DP	Phytase	50 PU
Cellulase blend	200 CU	Pectinase	50 AJDU

Helpful Ingredients:

Xylanase	L. acidophilus
Beta-glucanase	L. bifidus
Hemicellulase	

*High Cellulase Formula three times a day between meals for one to two weeks

Purpose: To manage yeast overgrowth
Each capsule should contain approximately:

Cellulase blend	30,000 CU
Protease blend	100,000 HUT

Contraindications: High amounts of cellulase should not be taken with certain timed-release medications that contain cellulose.

*Probiotic Formula two times daily on an empty stomach for one month, then daily before bed

Purpose: To assist the body in balancing microflora
Each serving should contain approximately 5 billion probiotic live cells (guaranteed potency), comprised of:

Bacillus Subtillis	No less than 3 billion CFU guaranteed potency	A blend of L. acidophilus, L. casei, L. bulgaris, L. plantarum, L. rhamnosus, L. salivarius	No less than 1 billion CFU guaranteed potency
L. paracassei F-19	No less than 1 billion CFU guaranteed potency		

High Protease Formula three times daily between meals

Purpose: To help support immune function and assist in removing viruses, fungal forms, toxins, bacteria, and heavy metals
　　Each capsule should contain approximately:

Protease blend	150,000 HUT	Serratiopeptidase	25,000 units
Mucolase	8 mg	Nattokinase blend	400 FU
Catalase	50 baker units		

BAD BREATH

See HALITOSIS or PERIODONTAL DISORDERS.

BEDSORES

See SKIN ULCERS.

BLADDER INFECTION

The bladder is the hollow, muscular organ that acts as a reservoir for urine until it can be expelled from the body. Cystitis is a common infection of the bladder, most commonly affecting women. In the event of bladder discomfort or painful (frequent) urination, recommendations include a urinalysis to rule out infection, increased intake of fluids, acidifying the urine (as with cranberry juice), and supporting the immune system. Enzyme therapy can be used to improve the pH balance in the body to lower the chances or frequency of bladder infection, particularly if you are increasing intake of acidic foods or liquids, and to support the immune system. (See also KIDNEY STRESS.)

ENZYME SUPPLEMENTATION SUGGESTIONS:

*High Protease Formula three times daily between meals

Purpose: To help support immune function and assist in removing viruses, fungal forms, toxins, bacteria, and heavy metals
　　Each capsule should contain approximately:

Protease blend	150,000 HUT	Serratiopeptidase	25,000 units
Mucolase	8 mg	Nattokinase blend	400 FU
Catalase	50 baker units		

*pH Balancing Formula three times daily between meals

Purpose: To help the body achieve an optimal pH
  Each serving should contain approximately:

Amylase blend	25,000 DU	Lipase blend	175 FCCFIP
Cellulase blend	6,000 CU	Pectinase/Phytase	200 PU
Mineral blend	Potassium bicarbonate, sodium bicarbonate, magnesium citrate	Herbal blend	Hydrilla, marshmallow, papaya
Protease blend	1,000 HUT		

The formula should not exceed 8.0 on the pH scale and the capsule should be enteric coated.

High Potency Digestive Formula with every meal

Purpose: To radically enhance the digestion and assimilation of food while reducing the body's need to produce digestive enzymes; the higher potency formula will average about three times the potency of the average digestive formula; an average formula may be substituted if three times the regular dose is taken
  Each serving should contain approximately:

Amylase blend	22,000 DU	Alpha-galactosidase	450 GALU
Protease blend	80,000 HUT	Phytase	50 PU
Lipase blend	3,000 FCCFIP	Pectinase	50 AJDU
Cellulase blend	2,000 CU	Xylanase	500 XU
Invertase	80 IAU	Hemicellulase	30 HCU
Lactase	900 LacU	Beta-glucanase	25 BGU
Maltase	200 DP	L. acidophilus	250 million CFU
Glucoamylase	50 AGU		

Serratiopeptidase Formula

Purpose: To break down protein and reduce inflammation. Also supports cardiovascular health and enhances other proteases.
  Each serving should contain approximately:

Serratiopeptidase	80,000 SU
Protease blend	70,000 HUT
Mineral blend	50 mg

Supporting enzymes:

Bromelain	Papain

BLOOD CLEANSE

The blood's main function is to act as a transport system, but it also plays a major role in the defense against infection. White blood cells are our defense against infection by viruses, bacteria, fungi, and parasites, as well as any inflammation (refer to chapter 3). Hemoglobin, a protein present in red blood cells, helps carry oxygen from the lungs to the tissues, where it is exchanged for carbon dioxide. Almost half the volume of blood consists of red and white blood cells, while the remainder is a fluid called plasma, which contains dissolved proteins, sugars, fats, and minerals. The protease in the high protease enzyme formula fortifies and cleanses the blood by helping to build the immune system and break down unwanted proteins in the blood. The pH balancing formula helps the body maintain a healthy pH balance in all systems, including the blood (see chapter 3). You should follow the regimen below for no less than one month, and ideally for nine weeks.

ENZYME SUPPLEMENTATION SUGGESTIONS:

*High Potency Digestive Formula with every meal

Purpose: To radically enhance the digestion and assimilation of food while reducing the body's need to produce digestive enzymes; the higher potency formula will average about three times the potency of the average digestive formula; an average formula may be substituted if three times the regular dose is taken
Each serving should contain approximately:

Amylase blend	22,000 DU	Alpha-galactosidase	450 GALU
Protease blend	80,000 HUT	Phytase	50 PU
Lipase blend	3,000 FCCFIP	Pectinase	50 AJDU
Cellulase blend	2,000 CU	Xylanase	500 XU
Invertase	80 IAU	Hemicellulase	30 HCU
Lactase	900 LacU	Beta-glucanase	25 BGU
Maltase	200 DP	L. acidophilus	250 million CFU
Glucoamylase	50 AGU		

*High Protease Formula three times daily between meals

Purpose: To help support immune function and assist in removing viruses, fungal forms, toxins, bacteria, and heavy metals
Each capsule should contain approximately:

Protease blend	150,000 HUT	Serratiopeptidase	25,000 units
Mucolase	8 mg	Nattokinase blend	400 FU
Catalase	50 baker units		

pH Balancing Formula three times daily between meals

Purpose: To help the body achieve an optimal pH
Each serving should contain approximately:

Amylase blend	25,000 DU	Lipase blend	175 FCCFIP
Cellulase blend	6,000 CU	Pectinase/Phytase	200 PU
Mineral blend	Potassium bicarbonate, sodium bicarbonate, magnesium citrate	Herbal blend	Hydrilla, marshmallow, papaya
Protease blend	1,000 HUT		

The formula should not exceed 8.0 on the pH scale and the capsule should be enteric coated.

BONE FRACTURES

A fracture is a break in a bone that can be either simple or compound. Compound fractures break through the skin, presenting increased risk of infection due to exposure to bacteria and other harmful elements. All fractures must be treated by a doctor and will, at the least, require immobilization of the affected area with a cast. Some forms of fractures will require surgery.

Enzymes can be used to support the body's ability to heal the bone and the surrounding tissue after a doctor has seen to it and ward off infection or other associated problems by optimizing digestion to improve nutrient absorption, reducing inflammation, and eliminating or reducing the risk of blood clots. The addition of mineral supplements to aid in bone and tissue regeneration would also be beneficial.

ENZYME SUPPLEMENTATION SUGGESTIONS:

*High Potency Digestive Formula** with every meal

Purpose: To radically enhance the digestion and assimilation of food while reducing the body's need to produce digestive enzymes; the higher potency formula will average about three times the potency of the average digestive formula; an average formula may be substituted if three times the regular dose is taken
   Each serving should contain approximately:

Amylase blend	22,000 DU	Alpha-galactosidase	450 GALU
Protease blend	80,000 HUT	Phytase	50 PU
Lipase blend	3,000 FCCFIP	Pectinase	50 AJDU
Cellulase blend	2,000 CU	Xylanase	500 XU
Invertase	80 IAU	Hemicellulase	30 HCU
Lactase	900 LacU	Beta-glucanase	25 BGU
Maltase	200 DP	L. acidophilus	250 million CFU
Glucoamylase	50 AGU		

*Anti-inflammatory Formula** three times daily (more may be taken as needed)

Purpose: To address inflammation, speed recovery, and repair tissue; best if enteric coated
   Each serving should contain approximately:

Protease blend	120,000 HUT	Amylase blend	7,000 DU
Papain	140,000 PU	Lipase blend	600 FCCFIP
Bromelain	1,200 GDU (11.25 million FCCPU)	Catalase	100 baker units

Serratiopeptidase Formula may be added to the anti-inflammatory enzyme formula for chronic pain

Purpose: To break down protein and reduce inflammation. Also supports cardiovascular health and enhances other proteases.
   Each serving should contain approximately:

Serratiopeptidase	80,000 SU
Protease blend	70,000 HUT
Mineral blend	50 mg

Supporting enzymes:

Bromelain	Papain

BRONCHITIS

Both bacteria and viruses can cause bronchitis, an inflammation of the bronchi (the airways that connect the trachea to the lungs). Chronic bronchitis typically results from repeated lung irritation and may be caused by allergies, smoking, and regular exposure to heavy atmospheric pollution. Those who suffer from chronic bronchitis have a higher risk of developing heart disease. Acute bronchitis generally develops following upper respiratory tract infections and can develop into pneumonia. Symptoms of bronchitis can include difficulty breathing, fever, sore throat, a mucous build-up, and coughing.

It is important to consult a physician to determine the underlying cause of the condition. Enzyme therapy can be used to reduce congestion and inflammation and support the digestive and immune systems.

ENZYME SUPPLEMENTATION SUGGESTIONS:
*Mucolase Formula three times daily between meals

Purpose: To reduce excess mucus produced by the body; particularly helpful in treating sinus and chest congestion
Each serving should contain approximately:

Mucolase	30 mg

Supporting enzymes:

Amylase blend	7,000 DU	Cellulase blend	200 CU
Protease blend	20,000 HUT	Xylanase	250 XU
Glucoamylase	25 AGU	Pectinase with Phytase	175 endo-PG
Beta-glucanase	30 BGU	Hemicellulase	30 HCU
Lipase blend	250 FCCFIP	Invertase	5 INVU
Alpha-galactosidase	50 GALU		

*High Protease Formula three times daily between meals

Purpose: To help support immune function and assist in removing viruses, fungal forms, toxins, bacteria, and heavy metals
Each capsule should contain approximately:

Protease blend	150,000 HUT	Serratiopeptidase	25,000 units
Mucolase	8 mg	Nattokinase blend	400 FU
Catalase	50 baker units		

High Potency Digestive Formula with every meal

Purpose: To radically enhance the digestion and assimilation of food while reducing the body's need to produce digestive enzymes; the higher potency formula will average about three times the potency of the average digestive formula; an average formula may be substituted if three times the regular dose is taken

Each serving should contain approximately:

Amylase blend	22,000 DU	Alpha-galactosidase	450 GALU
Protease blend	80,000 HUT	Phytase	50 PU
Lipase blend	3,000 FCCFIP	Pectinase	50 AJDU
Cellulase blend	2,000 CU	Xylanase	500 XU
Invertase	80 IAU	Hemicellulase	30 HCU
Lactase	900 LacU	Beta-glucanase	25 BGU
Maltase	200 DP	L. acidophilus	250 million CFU
Glucoamylase	50 AGU		

BRUISING

See SPORTS INJURIES.

BURSITIS

Bursitis is characterized by inflammation of, tenderness of, and fluid accumulation in the bursae (flat, sac-like membranes), which protect the tendons, muscles, and bones from friction. This condition may result from injury, strain, infection, calcium deposits, or arthritis. Often acute pain limits the range of motion of the affected joint. The lower knee, hip, shoulder, and elbow are the most common locations of inflammation.

Recommendations for treatment include resting the joint, compression of the area and ice to limit swelling, and elevation of the injured area to encourage the drainage of fluids. Enzymes can be used to support nutrient absorption, reduce inflammation, and speed healing.

ENZYME SUPPLEMENTATION SUGGESTIONS:

*High Potency Digestive Formula with every meal

Purpose: To radically enhance the digestion and assimilation of food while reducing the body's need to produce digestive enzymes; the higher potency formula will average about three times the potency of the average digestive formula; an average formula may be substituted if three times the regular dose is taken
Each serving should contain approximately:

Amylase blend	22,000 DU	Alpha-galactosidase	450 GALU
Protease blend	80,000 HUT	Phytase	50 PU
Lipase blend	3,000 FCCFIP	Pectinase	50 AJDU
Cellulase blend	2,000 CU	Xylanase	500 XU
Invertase	80 IAU	Hemicellulase	30 HCU
Lactase	900 LacU	Beta-glucanase	25 BGU
Maltase	200 DP	L. acidophilus	250 million CFU
Glucoamylase	50 AGU		

*Anti-inflammatory Formula three times daily; more may be taken as needed

Purpose: To address inflammation, speed recovery, and repair tissue; best if enteric coated
Each serving should contain approximately:

Protease blend	120,000 HUT	Amylase blend	7,000 DU
Papain	140,000 PU	Lipase blend	600 FCCFIP
Bromelain	1,200 GDU (11.25 million FCCPU)	Catalase	100 baker units

High Protease Formula or Nattokinase Formula three times daily

Purpose: To help support immune function and assist in removing viruses, fungal forms, toxins, bacteria, and heavy metals
Each capsule should contain approximately:

Protease blend	150,000 HUT	Serratiopeptidase	25,000 units
Mucolase	8 mg	Nattokinase blend	400 FU
Catalase	50 baker units		

Purpose: To support cardiovascular health and decrease blood pressure by breaking down fibrin

Each serving should contain approximately:

Necessary ingredient:

Nattokinase NSK-SD	1,000 FU

Helpful ingredients:

Amylase blend	9,000 DU	Glucoamylase	25 AGU
Protease blend	20,000 HUT	Lipase blend	1,000 FCCFIP
Minerals	85 mg	Cellulase blend	400 CU

Optional: Serratiopeptidase Formula may be added for chronic pain relief.

Purpose: To break down protein and reduce inflammation. Also supports cardiovascular health and enhances other proteases.

Each serving should contain approximately:

Serratiopeptidase	80,000 SU
Protease blend	70,000 HUT
Mineral blend	50 mg

Supporting enzymes:

Bromelain	Papain

CANCER

Over one hundred types of cancer have been discovered, all with different causes and rates of aggression. Research indicates that some contributing factors include inflammation, stress, poor diet, hereditary and environmental factors, exposure to certain toxins and chemicals, and a compromised immune system, although specific causes of individual types of cancer or tumors have not been identified. The development of cancer begins with initiation, which is the process of genetic change within a cell that makes it possible for the cell to become cancerous. The development continues with promotion, which allows the cancerous cell to grow into a tumor. Cancerous cells can avoid detection, and therefore elimination, by the body's immune system. There are five categories of cancer: Sarcomas affect the connective tissue, muscles, and bones; carcinomas affect the skin, glands, organs, and mucous membranes; lymphomas affect the lymphatic system; leukemias affect the blood; and myelomas, which are very rare, affect the plasma of the bone marrow.

Many different forms of treatment are available depending on the type of cancer, including chemotherapy, drugs, radiation, nutritional support, and immune system stimulation and support. Because there are so many different types of cancer, all requiring different types of intervention, individuals must work with an oncologist to determine the best course of therapy, including the use of enzyme therapies.

Enzymes are the basis for certain anticancer drugs, but separate enzyme therapy has also been studied in cancer patients. Enzyme therapy has been shown to reduce the instance or risk of metastasis and to help patients with leukemia better tolerate chemotherapy ("Enzyme Makes Chemo More Tolerable," Roswell Park Cancer Institute Dept. of Epidemiology, April 16 2007, newswise.com). Enzyme therapy can be used in a more general way to support the absorption of nutrients, strengthen the immune system, reduce inflammation, prevent thrombosis, increase circulation, and balance the body's systems to promote better overall health and conserve energy to fight the cancer.

ENZYME SUPPLEMENTATION SUGGESTIONS:

*High Potency Digestive Formula with every meal

Purpose: To radically enhance the digestion and assimilation of food while reducing the body's need to produce digestive enzymes; the higher potency formula will average about three times the potency of the average digestive formula; an average formula may be substituted if three times the regular dose is taken
   Each serving should contain approximately:

Amylase blend	22,000 DU	Alpha-galactosidase	450 GALU
Protease blend	80,000 HUT	Phytase	50 PU
Lipase blend	3,000 FCCFIP	Pectinase	50 AJDU
Cellulase blend	2,000 CU	Xylanase	500 XU
Invertase	80 IAU	Hemicellulase	30 HCU
Lactase	900 LacU	Beta-glucanase	25 BGU
Maltase	200 DP	L. acidophilus	250 million CFU
Glucoamylase	50 AGU		

*High Protease Formula at least three times daily

Purpose: To help support immune function and assist in removing viruses, fungal forms, toxins, bacteria, and heavy metals
Each capsule should contain approximately:

Protease blend	150,000 HUT	Serratiopeptidase	25,000 units
Mucolase	8 mg	Nattokinase blend	400 FU
Catalase	50 baker units		

*Nattokinase Formula three times a day between meals

Purpose: To increase circulation and break down fibrin
Each serving should contain approximately:
Necessary ingredient:

Nattokinase NSK-SD	1,000 FU

Helpful ingredients:

Amylase blend	9,000 DU	Glucoamylase	25 AGU
Protease blend	20,000 HUT	Lipase blend	1,000 FCCFIP
Minerals	85 mg	Cellulase blend	400 CU

*pH Balancing Formula four times per day between meals

Purpose: To help the body achieve an optimal pH
Each serving should contain approximately:

Amylase blend	25,000 DU	Lipase blend	175 FCCFIP
Cellulase blend	6,000 CU	Pectinase/Phytase	200 PU
Mineral blend	Potassium bicarbonate, sodium bicarbonate, magnesium citrate	Herbal blend	Hydrilla, marshmallow, papaya
Protease blend	1,000 HUT		

The formula should not exceed 8.0 on the pH scale and the capsule should be enteric coated.

Probiotic Formula daily

Purpose: To assist the body in balancing microflora

Each serving should contain approximately 5 billion probiotic live cells (guaranteed potency), comprised of:

Bacillus Subtillis	No less than 3 billion CFU guaranteed potency	A blend of *L. acidophilus, L. casei, L. bulgaris, L. plantarum, L. rhamnosus, L. salivarius*	No less than 1 billion CFU guaranteed potency
L. paracassei F-19	No less than 1 billion CFU guaranteed potency		

Optional: Anti-inflammatory Formula may be added for pain or inflammation

Purpose: To address inflammation, speed recovery, and repair tissue; best if enteric coated
Each serving should contain approximately:

Protease blend	120,000 HUT	Amylase blend	7,000 DU
Papain	140,000 PU	Lipase blend	600 FCCFIP
Bromelain	1,200 GDU (11.25 million FCCPU)	Catalase	100 baker units

CANDIDIASIS

This condition involves the overgrowth of the fungus *Candida albicans*, which normally exists in an ecological equilibrium throughout the body. (See chapter 3.) Under certain conditions this fungus proliferates, weakening the immune system, causing infections, and leading to a wide host of symptoms, including thrush (yeast infection of the mouth), yeast infection of the vagina, depression, congestion, digestive tract disturbances, acne, muscle and joint pain, heightened environmental sensitivities, hypothyroidism, and adrenal insufficiencies. Individuals who may have a higher risk of developing yeast infections include diabetics, those suffering from chronic diseases, individuals who are obese, those who take antibiotics, and oral contraceptive users. The use of antibiotics, nutrient and digestive deficiencies, altered bowel flora, and impaired liver function can also contribute to *Candida* overgrowth.

Recommendations include identifying predisposing factors and following a *Candida* control diet (low in sugar, simple carbohydrates, and alcohol). This promotes effective detoxification and elimination. It is also important to support the digestive and immune systems. Enzymes can be used to help achieve these goals and to balance other systems in the body to ensure overall health.

ENZYME SUPPLEMENTATION SUGGESTIONS:

*High Cellulase Formula three times daily between meals for two weeks

Purpose: To manage yeast overgrowth
    Each capsule should contain approximately:

Cellulase blend	30,000 CU
Protease blend	100,000 HUT

Contraindications: High amounts of cellulase should not be taken with certain timed-release medications that contain cellulose.

*High Protease Formula added in acute or chronic conditions

Purpose: To help support immune function and assist in removing viruses, fungal forms, toxins, bacteria, and heavy metals
    Each capsule should contain approximately:

Protease blend	150,000 HUT	Serratiopeptidase	25,000 units
Mucolase	8 mg	Nattokinase blend	400 FU
Catalase	50 baker units		

*Probiotic Formula daily before bed

Purpose: To assist the body in balancing microflora
    Each serving should contain approximately 5 billion probiotic live cells (guaranteed potency), comprised of:

Bacillus Subtillis	No less than 3 billion CFU guaranteed potency	A blend of *L. acidophilus, L. casei, L. bulgaris, L. plantarum, L. rhamnosus, L. salivarius*	No less than 1 billion CFU guaranteed potency
L. paracassei F-19	No less than 1 billion CFU guaranteed potency		

High Potency Digestive Formula with every meal

Purpose: To radically enhance the digestion and assimilation of food while reducing the body's need to produce digestive enzymes; the higher potency formula will average about three times the potency of the average digestive formula; an average formula may be substituted if three times the regular dose is taken

Each serving should contain approximately:

Amylase blend	22,000 DU	Alpha-galactosidase	450 GALU
Protease blend	80,000 HUT	Phytase	50 PU
Lipase blend	3,000 FCCFIP	Pectinase	50 AJDU
Cellulase blend	2,000 CU	Xylanase	500 XU
Invertase	80 IAU	Hemicellulase	30 HCU
Lactase	900 LacU	Beta-glucanase	25 BGU
Maltase	200 DP	L. acidophilus	250 million CFU
Glucoamylase	50 AGU		

High Amylase Formula may be added any time to increase energy level

Purpose: To overcome symptoms of allergies and for the proper digestion of carbohydrates, especially grains, raw vegetables, and legumes
Each serving should contain approximately:

Amylase blend	22,000 DU	Cellulase blend	400 CU
Glucoamylase	30 AGU	Lactase	300 LacU
Alpha-galactosidase	1,000 GALU	Maltase	300 DP
Protease blend	15,000 HUT	Pectinase	20 endo-PG
Lipase blend	150 FCCFIP		

Optional: pH Balancing Formula two times daily

Purpose: To help the body achieve an optimal pH
Each serving should contain approximately:

Amylase blend	25,000 DU	Lipase blend	175 FCCFIP
Cellulase blend	6,000 CU	Pectinase/Phytase	200 PU
Mineral blend	Potassium bicarbonate, sodium bicarbonate, magnesium citrate	Herbal blend	Hydrilla, marshmallow, papaya
Protease blend	1,000 HUT		

The formula should not exceed 8.0 on the pH scale and the capsule should be enteric coated.

CANKER SORES

Canker sores (aphthous ulcers) are painful, persistent, and annoying sores on or under the tongue, on the soft palate, on the inside of the cheeks or lips, or at the base of the gums. The sores can range from the size of a pinhead to the size of a quarter, but they are not contagious. Canker sores are different from fever blisters or cold sores, which are caused by the herpes virus and are contagious. Fever blisters are usually found on the outside of the lips or on the corners of the mouth.

Recurrent canker sores appear to be related to stress, nutrient deficiencies, hormonal imbalances, poor dental hygiene, Crohn's Disease or other digestive tract ailments, and food sensitivities (particularly to gluten, milk, and chocolate).

Recommendations include reducing stress, eliminating food allergens, and correcting nutrient deficiencies to balance the body's minerals and pH. A B-vitamin complex has also been shown to be beneficial. Enzymes can be used to support improved nutrient absorption, balance the body's pH, and support the immune system.

ENZYME SUPPLEMENTATION SUGGESTIONS:
*Probiotic Formula two times a day on an empty stomach

Purpose: To assist the body in balancing microflora
Each serving should contain approximately 5 billion probiotic live cells (guaranteed potency), comprised of:

Bacillus Subtillis	No less than 3 billion CFU guaranteed potency	A blend of *L. acidophilus, L. casei, L. bulgaris, L. plantarum, L. rhamnosus, L. salivarius*	No less than 1 billion CFU guaranteed potency
L. paracassei F-19	No less than 1 billion CFU guaranteed potency		

*pH Balancing Formula two times per day between meals

Purpose: To help the body achieve an optimal pH
Each serving should contain approximately:

Amylase blend	25,000 DU	Lipase blend	175 FCCFIP
Cellulase blend	6,000 CU	Pectinase/Phytase	200 PU
Mineral blend	Potassium bicarbonate, sodium bicarbonate, magnesium citrate	Herbal blend	Hydrilla, marshmallow, papaya
Protease blend	1,000 HUT		

The formula should not exceed 8.0 on the pH scale and the capsule should be enteric coated.

High Potency Digestive Formula with every meal

Purpose: To radically enhance the digestion and assimilation of food while reducing the body's need to produce digestive enzymes; the higher potency formula will average about three times the potency of the average digestive formula; an average formula may be substituted if three times the regular dose is taken

Each serving should contain approximately:

Amylase blend	22,000 DU	Alpha-galactosidase	450 GALU
Protease blend	80,000 HUT	Phytase	50 PU
Lipase blend	3,000 FCCFIP	Pectinase	50 AJDU
Cellulase blend	2,000 CU	Xylanase	500 XU
Invertase	80 IAU	Hemicellulase	30 HCU
Lactase	900 LacU	Beta-glucanase	25 BGU
Maltase	200 DP	L. acidophilus	250 million CFU
Glucoamylase	50 AGU		

High Protease Formula added before, during, and after breakout

Purpose: To help support immune function and assist in removing viruses, fungal forms, toxins, bacteria, and heavy metals

Each capsule should contain approximately:

Protease blend	150,000 HUT	Serratiopeptidase	25,000 units
Mucolase	8 mg	Nattokinase blend	400 FU
Catalase	50 baker units		

CELIAC DISEASE

This rare genetic disorder is characterized by an allergic reaction to gluten. The body reacts to ingested gluten by releasing antibodies. Over time, these antibodies damage the lining of the small intestine, causing an abnormal structure. This results in an impaired ability to absorb vitamins and minerals, or malabsorption. Malabsorption generally becomes a serious problem. A diagnosis of celiac disease is confirmed by a biopsy of the small intestine.

Symptoms of celiac disease include diarrhea, nausea, abdominal swelling, foul-smelling greasy stools, weight loss, anemia, joint or bone pain, and skin rashes. Dietary recommendations include eliminating of foods containing gluten or milk products.

Studies have shown that high percentages of people with moderate to severe celiac disease are deficient in digestive enzymes because of damage to the lining of the small intestine (G. M. Gray, "Disaccharidases of the Small Intestine in Selected Diseases," in D. D. Katz (ed.), *Human Health and Disease,* (Bethesda, MD: FASEB

1980): 124.). Therefore, a high potency digestive enzyme supplement can be very beneficial. In addition, enzymes can be used to support the body's immune system, pH balance, and microflora balance, all of which may be suffering.

ENZYME SUPPLEMENTATION SUGGESTIONS:

*High Potency Digestive Formula with every meal

Purpose: To radically enhance the digestion and assimilation of food while reducing the body's need to produce digestive enzymes; the higher potency formula will average about three times the potency of the average digestive formula; an average formula may be substituted if three times the regular dose is taken

Each serving should contain approximately:

Amylase blend	22,000 DU	Alpha-galactosidase	450 GALU
Protease blend	80,000 HUT	Phytase	50 PU
Lipase blend	3,000 FCCFIP	Pectinase	50 AJDU
Cellulase blend	2,000 CU	Xylanase	500 XU
Invertase	80 IAU	Hemicellulase	30 HCU
Lactase	900 LacU	Beta-glucanase	25 BGU
Maltase	200 DP	L. acidophilus	250 million CFU
Glucoamylase	50 AGU		

*DPPIV Formula whenever foods containing gluten are eaten or there is potential that foods eaten have been cooked with foods containing gluten (such as when eating out)

Purpose: To digest gluten (a common allergen found in wheat and cereal grains). DPPIV has proven helpful for individuals who are sensitive to gluten.

Each serving should contain approximately:

DPPIV Protease blend	80,000 HUT	Glucoamylase	15,000 AGU
Amylase blend	15,000 DU		

*Probiotic Formula daily

Purpose: To assist the body in balancing microflora

Each serving should contain approximately 5 billion probiotic live cells (guaranteed potency), comprised of:

Bacillus Subtillis	No less than 3 billion CFU guaranteed potency	A blend of L. acidophilus, L. casei, L. bulgaris, L. plantarum, L. rhamnosus, L. salivarius	No less than 1 billion CFU guaranteed potency
L. paracassei F-19	No less than 1 billion CFU guaranteed potency		

High Protease Formula three times daily between meals

Purpose: To help support immune function and assist in removing viruses, fungal forms, toxins, bacteria, and heavy metals

Each capsule should contain approximately:

Protease blend	150,000 HUT	Serratiopeptidase	25,000 units
Mucolase	8 mg	Nattokinase blend	400 FU
Catalase	50 baker units		

High Cellulase Formula three times daily between meals for one week

Purpose: To manage yeast overgrowth

Each capsule should contain approximately:

Cellulase blend	30,000 CU
Protease blend	100,000 HUT

Contraindications: High amounts of cellulase should not be taken with certain timed-release medications that contain cellulose.

Soothing Digestive Formula as needed for nausea or intestinal inflammation

Purpose: To help alleviate conditions associated with gastrointestinal distress

Each serving should contain approximately:

Amylase blend	2,000 DU	Gotu kola	50 mg
Lipase blend	175 FCCFIP	Papaya leaf	100 mg
Cellulase blend	400 CU	Prickly ash bark	50 mg
Marshmallow root	100 mg		

Additional helpful ingredients:

DGL (deglycyrrhizinated licorice)	

This formula should *not* contain protease. Other herbs may also be present.

Optional: pH Balancing Formula three times daily

Purpose: To help the body achieve an optimal pH
    Each serving should contain approximately:

Amylase blend	25,000 DU	Lipase blend	175 FCCFIP
Cellulase blend	6,000 CU	Pectinase/Phytase	200 PU
Mineral blend	Potassium bicarbonate, sodium bicarbonate, magnesium citrate	Herbal blend	Hydrilla, marshmallow, papaya
Protease blend	1,000 HUT		

The formula should not exceed 8.0 on the pH scale and the capsule should be enteric coated.

CHOLESTEROL (ELEVATED)

Cholesterol is a waxy substance produced by the liver and absorbed from certain foods. It is an important constituent of body cells, important for proper nerve and brain function, and a necessary element in the formation of hormones and in the transport of cholesterol in the bloodstream back to the liver. But high blood cholesterol can cause fatty tissue to accumulate on the inner lining of arteries, which often results in heart disease or strokes. Diet, heredity, and metabolic diseases influence the level of cholesterol in the blood.

There are two components to cholesterol: LDL (low-density lipoprotein) and HDL (high-density lipoprotein). HDLs are often called "good cholesterol" because they perform key functions in the body. LDLs are often called "bad cholesterol" because when they are elevated, they collect on the inside of blood vessel walls, potentially leading to blocked blood vessels, heart disease, and stroke.

Recommendations for treating high cholesterol include a well-balanced, low-fat (not nonfat), low-sugar diet; daily exercise; supplemental nutrients to elevate HDL levels; and regular monitoring of the cholesterol levels. Enzymes can help support health by improving digestion and proper absorption and elimination of fats and sugars and by improving the health of blood vessels and the heart.

ENZYME SUPPLEMENTATION SUGGESTIONS:

*High Lipase Enzyme Formula three times daily between meals

Purpose: To improve fat digestion and metabolism, as well as the health of the cardio-vascular system

Each capsule should contain approximately:

Lipase blend	5,000 FCCFIP	Protease blend	20,000 HUT
Amylase blend	10,000 DU	Lactase	300 LacU

*Nattokinase Formula three times daily (for heart health)

Purpose: To support cardiovascular health and decrease blood pressure by breaking down fibrin
Each serving should contain approximately:
Necessary ingredient:

Nattokinase NSK-SD	1,000 FU

Helpful ingredients:

Amylase blend	9,000 DU	Glucoamylase	25 AGU
Protease blend	20,000 HUT	Lipase blend	1,000 FCCFIP
Minerals	85 mg	Cellulase blend	400 CU

High Potency Digestive Enzyme Formula or High Amylase Digestion Formula with every meal (for compete breakdown of sugars)

Purpose: To radically enhance the digestion and assimilation of food while reducing the body's need to produce digestive enzymes; the higher potency formula will average about three times the potency of the average digestive formula; an average formula may be substituted if three times the regular dose is taken
Each serving should contain approximately:

Amylase blend	22,000 DU	Alpha-galactosidase	450 GALU
Protease blend	80,000 HUT	Phytase	50 PU
Lipase blend	3,000 FCCFIP	Pectinase	50 AJDU
Cellulase blend	2,000 CU	Xylanase	500 XU
Invertase	80 IAU	Hemicellulase	30 HCU
Lactase	900 LacU	Beta-glucanase	25 BGU
Maltase	200 DP	L. acidophilus	250 million CFU
Glucoamylase	50 AGU		

Purpose: To overcome symptoms of allergies and for the proper digestion of carbohydrates, especially grains, raw vegetables, and legumes
Each serving should contain approximately:

Amylase blend	22,000 DU	Cellulase blend	400 CU
Glucoamylase	30 AGU	Lactase	300 LacU
Alpha-galactosidase	1,000 GALU	Maltase	300 DP
Protease blend	15,000 HUT	Pectinase	20 endo-PG
Lipase blend	150 FCCFIP		

CHRONIC FATIGUE SYNDROME

Chronic fatigue syndrome (CFS) is a condition with a variety of symptoms, the most dominant being debilitating, persistent fatigue. Diagnosing CFS can be difficult because the symptoms are so varied and because, individually, none of them may be severe. Sometimes the person with CFS doesn't even feel physically ill enough to seek professional help. Individuals are typically diagnosed with CFS when they exhibit patterns of the most common symptoms continuously within a six-month period. A common belief that weaves throughout all of the research is that people who develop CFS have a genetic predisposition for this syndrome. In 1999, research showed that more than five million people in the United States have been diagnosed with CFS. There are likely many more who have not been properly diagnosed.

CFS is closely related to fibromyalgia (see FIBROMYALGIA), and shares many common symptoms. Research indicates that people with CFS or fibromyalgia have defects in the neuroregulatory system, which results in abnormal production of neurotransmitters, such as seratonin, melatonin, dopamine, and other chemicals that help control pain, mood, sleep, and the immune system. This is the reason for the wide array of symptoms associated with this condition. The symptoms of CFS and fibromyalgia may include sore throat, low-grade fever, recurrent fatigue, headaches, lymph node swelling, intestinal discomfort, digestive difficulties, emotional stress, depression, and muscle and joint pain. Many people also experience severe stress and depression. Those who suffer from CFS or fibromyalgia often do not look sick, so they find themselves constantly on the defensive with their family and friends. The primary difference between CFS and fibromyalgia is that CFS has the diagnostic requirement of fatigue and fibromyalgia has the requirement of musculoskeletal pain.

Research shows that people with CFS or fibromyalgia experience a lack of the polysaccharolytic enzymes early in life. Polysaccharolytic enzymes are the catalysts that break down carbohydrates. Clinically, it is shown that people with fibromyalgia or CFS have digestive problems with carbohydrates (starches). Many also have a lipase deficiency. Lack of the proper lipolytic enzymes results in fatty acid imbalances and possibly hormonal imbalances.

Some of the latest information on CFS comes from the Temple University School of Medicine in Philadelphia. Dr. Suhadolnik, a professor of biochemistry and a member of the university's Institute of Cancer Research and Molecular Biology, explains, "All CFS patients tested have a new enzyme, while none of the healthy controls do." This newly discovered enzyme is suspected to be inferior to the enzyme that people who do not suffer from CFS have. He feels this explains why CFS patients have a hard time maintaining the energy for cellular growth.

Successfully treating CFS requires a comprehensive approach to identifying the underlying causative factors. Recommendations include lifestyle modification to reduce and manage stress, identification of food allergies, counseling, daily exercise, detoxification, and optimum support of the digestive and immune systems. Enzyme therapy can improve digestion and absorption of nutrients, help strengthen the immune system, balance the body's pH, and fight inflammation and symptoms of allergic responses.

ENZYME SUPPLEMENTATION SUGGESTIONS:

*High Potency Digestive Formula (add Soothing Digestive Formula if necessary)

Purpose: To radically enhance the digestion and assimilation of food while reducing the body's need to produce digestive enzymes; the higher potency formula will average about three times the potency of the average digestive formula; an average formula may be substituted if three times the regular dose is taken

Each serving should contain approximately:

Amylase blend	22,000 DU	Alpha-galactosidase	450 GALU
Protease blend	80,000 HUT	Phytase	50 PU
Lipase blend	3,000 FCCFIP	Pectinase	50 AJDU
Cellulase blend	2,000 CU	Xylanase	500 XU
Invertase	80 IAU	Hemicellulase	30 HCU
Lactase	900 LacU	Beta-glucanase	25 BGU
Maltase	200 DP	L. acidophilus	250 million CFU
Glucoamylase	50 AGU		

*Anti-inflammatory Formula three times daily for inflammation (more or a serratiopeptidase enzyme formula may be added for pain)

Purpose: To address inflammation, speed recovery, and repair tissue; best if enteric coated
Each serving should contain approximately:

Protease blend	120,000 HUT	Amylase blend	7,000 DU
Papain	140,000 PU	Lipase blend	600 FCCFIP
Bromelain	1,200 GDU (11.25 million FCCPU)	Catalase	100 baker units

*High Protease Formula three times daily

Purpose: To help support immune function and assist in removing viruses, fungal forms, toxins, bacteria, and heavy metals
Each capsule should contain approximately:

Protease blend	150,000 HUT	Serratiopeptidase	25,000 units
Mucolase	8 mg	Nattokinase blend	400 FU
Catalase	50 baker units		

pH Balancing Formula three times daily

Purpose: To help the body achieve an optimal pH
Each serving should contain approximately:

Amylase blend	25,000 DU	Lipase blend	175 FCCFIP
Cellulase blend	6,000 CU	Pectinase/Phytase	200 PU
Mineral blend	Potassium bicarbonate, sodium bicarbonate, magnesium citrate	Herbal blend	Hydrilla, marshmallow, papaya
Protease blend	1,000 HUT		

The formula should not exceed 8.0 on the pH scale and the capsule should be enteric coated.

Optional: High Amylase Formula may be added any time to increase energy level

Purpose: To overcome symptoms of allergies and for the proper digestion of carbohydrates, especially grains, raw vegetables, and legumes

Each serving should contain approximately:

Amylase blend	22,000 DU	Cellulase blend	400 CU
Glucoamylase	30 AGU	Lactase	300 LacU
Alpha-galactosidase	1,000 GALU	Maltase	300 DP
Protease blend	15,000 HUT	Pectinase	20 endo-PG
Lipase blend	150 FCCFIP		

CIRCULATION (POOR)

The continuous flow of blood throughout the body provides all tissues with a regular supply of oxygen and nutrients and carries away waste products. Poor circulation can result from a variety of conditions (varicose veins, arteriosclerosis, atherosclerosis, peripheral artery disease, diabetes) and can contribute to severe health issues, such as hypertension, heart attack, stroke, and gangrene. Therapeutic considerations for poor or restricted blood circulation should include daily exercise and using enzymes to support the digestive system and optimize the digestion and absorption of nutrients. Optimizing blood flow and maintaining the integrity of the cardiovascular system are essential, and enzyme therapy can support these goals.

ENZYME SUPPLEMENTATION SUGGESTIONS:

*High Potency Digestive Formula with every meal

Purpose: To radically enhance the digestion and assimilation of food while reducing the body's need to produce digestive enzymes; the higher potency formula will average about three times the potency of the average digestive formula; an average formula may be substituted if three times the regular dose is taken

Each serving should contain approximately:

Amylase blend	22,000 DU	Alpha-galactosidase	450 GALU
Protease blend	80,000 HUT	Phytase	50 PU
Lipase blend	3,000 FCCFIP	Pectinase	50 AJDU
Cellulase blend	2,000 CU	Xylanase	500 XU
Invertase	80 IAU	Hemicellulase	30 HCU
Lactase	900 LacU	Beta-glucanase	25 BGU
Maltase	200 DP	L. acidophilus	250 million CFU
Glucoamylase	50 AGU		

*Nattokinase Formula two times daily between meals

Purpose: To support cardiovascular health and decrease blood pressure by breaking down fibrin

Each serving should contain approximately:

Necessary ingredient:

Nattokinase NSK-SD	1,000 FU

Helpful ingredients:

Amylase blend	9,000 DU	Glucoamylase	25 AGU
Protease blend	20,000 HUT	Lipase blend	1,000 FCCFIP
Minerals	85 mg	Cellulase blend	400 CU

Optional: High Protease Formula may replace Nattokinase Formula

Purpose: To help support immune function and assist in removing viruses, fungal forms, toxins, bacteria, and heavy metals

Each capsule should contain approximately:

Protease blend	150,000 HUT	Serratiopeptidase	25,000 units
Mucolase	8 mg	Nattokinase blend	400 FU
Catalase	50 baker units		

COLDS

Almost two hundred viruses, all broadly similar, are known to cause colds. Symptoms of colds include sneezing, coughing, headache, fever, head congestion, restlessness, and generalized aches and pains. There are a variety of over-the-counter medications that can treat the symptoms of a cold, but none of them eliminate the cold virus. Enzyme therapy can support the functioning of the immune system and even introduce protease into the bloodstream to help attack the cold virus. Enzymes can also support the absorption of nutrients to improve overall health and help reduce the excess mucus being produced by the body.

ENZYME SUPPLEMENTATION SUGGESTIONS:

*High Protease Formula three to six times a day

Purpose: To help support immune function and assist in removing viruses, fungal forms, toxins, bacteria, and heavy metals

Each capsule should contain approximately:

Protease blend	150,000 HUT	Serratiopeptidase	25,000 units
Mucolase	8 mg	Nattokinase blend	400 FU
Catalase	50 baker units		

*Mucolase Formula three times daily between meals to address symptoms of congestion

Purpose: To reduce excess mucus produced by the body; particularly helpful in treating sinus and chest congestion
  Each serving should contain approximately:

Mucolase	30 mg

Supporting enzymes:

Amylase blend	7,000 DU	Cellulase blend	200 CU
Protease blend	20,000 HUT	Xylanase	250 XU
Glucoamylase	25 AGU	Pectinase with Phytase	175 endo-PG
Beta-glucanase	30 BGU	Hemicellulase	30 HCU
Lipase blend	250 FCCFIP	Invertase	5 INVU
Alpha-galactosidase	50 GALU		

High Potency Digestive Formula with every meal

Purpose: To radically enhance the digestion and assimilation of food while reducing the body's need to produce digestive enzymes; the higher potency formula will average about three times the potency of the average digestive formula; an average formula may be substituted if three times the regular dose is taken
  Each serving should contain approximately:

Amylase blend	22,000 DU	Alpha-galactosidase	450 GALU
Protease blend	80,000 HUT	Phytase	50 PU
Lipase blend	3,000 FCCFIP	Pectinase	50 AJDU
Cellulase blend	2,000 CU	Xylanase	500 XU
Invertase	80 IAU	Hemicellulase	30 HCU
Lactase	900 LacU	Beta-glucanase	25 BGU
Maltase	200 DP	L. acidophilus	250 million CFU
Glucoamylase	50 AGU		

COLIC (INFANTILE)

Colic is not a disease but a pattern of discomfort in infants typically associated with eating. The primary indicator of colic is excessive crying; the infant is typically inconsolable during bouts of colic. Colic is thought to be caused by spasms in the intestines of an infant, and may be triggered by a milk/dairy allergy or intolerance, but the research is not conclusive.

Infantile colic is common, occurring in approximately one in ten babies, starting between the first and sixth week of life and usually continuing until the child is three or four months old. The baby usually cries, turns red in the face, may pass gas, clench his fists, and draw up his legs. If the baby runs a fever or becomes ill with bouts of colic, a doctor should be consulted. Overstimulation, rapid environmental changes, and parents' anxiety will often make the child even more irritable.

Recommendations include creating a calm, quiet environment during and following mealtimes. Nursing mothers should not eat foods that may be contributing to gastrointestinal irritability in their infants, such as dairy products, onions, wheat, and broccoli. Administering digestive enzymes to the infant and mother before feeding times may also be highly beneficial.

ENZYME SUPPLEMENTATION SUGGESTIONS:

Infants: A half a capsule of digestive formula mixed in tepid water administered through a syringe or dropper into the child's mouth with every meal or bottle. If results are not satisfactory, increase dosage or repeat as often as needed. IMPORTANT NOTE: *Do not mix enzymes with breast milk or formula, since the enzymes will begin to hydrolyze it. Administer enzymes in water to the infant before the child ingests any food.*

Nursing Mothers: High Potency Digestive Formula with meals and before feedings.

Purpose: To radically enhance the digestion and assimilation of food while reducing the body's need to produce digestive enzymes; the higher potency formula will average about three times the potency of the average digestive formula; an average formula may be substituted if three times the regular dose is taken

Each serving should contain approximately:

Amylase blend	22,000 DU	Alpha-galactosidase	450 GALU
Protease blend	80,000 HUT	Phytase	50 PU
Lipase blend	3,000 FCCFIP	Pectinase	50 AJDU
Cellulase blend	2,000 CU	Xylanase	500 XU
Invertase	80 IAU	Hemicellulase	30 HCU
Lactase	900 LacU	Beta-glucanase	25 BGU
Maltase	200 DP	*L. acidophilus*	250 million CFU
Glucoamylase	50 AGU		

Rashes: If a rash develops, the mother should add a **High Cellulase Formula** three times per day to her diet.

Purpose: To manage yeast overgrowth
Each capsule should contain approximately:

Cellulase blend	30,000 CU
Protease blend	100,000 HUT

Contraindications: High amounts of cellulase should not be taken with certain timed-release medications that contain cellulose.

Infants: Dissolve 1/3 of **Digestive Formula** capsule and administer to infant before feeding.

Purpose: To enhance the digestion and assimilation of food while reducing the body's need to produce digestive enzymes
Each serving should contain approximately:
Necessary Ingredients:

Amylase blend	12,000 DU	Alpha-galactosidase	75 GALU
Protease blend	42,000 HUT	Lipase blend	500 FCCFIP
Invertase	10 IAU	Lactase	850 LacU
Maltase	200 DP	Phytase	50 PU
Cellulase blend	200 CU	Pectinase	50 AJDU

Helpful Ingredients:

Xylanase	L. acidophilus
Beta-glucanase	L. bifidus
Hemicellulase	

COLITIS, ULCERATIVE

See INFLAMMATORY BOWEL DISEASE.

CONSTIPATION

Constipation is the infrequent or difficult passing of hard, dry feces. It is important that the bowels move daily. Harmful toxins can build up as a result of waste products that remain in the colon for longer than four hours. Constipation increases the risk of other difficulties, including indigestion, hemorrhoids, piles, obesity, diverticulitis, appendicitis, hernias, and cancer.

Recommendations include increasing hydration, increasing fiber in the diet, regular exercise, and digestive enzyme and probiotic supplements to enhance digestion and absorption of nutrients to maintain healthy intestinal flora.

ENZYME SUPPLEMENTATION SUGGESTIONS:

*High Potency Digestive Formula with every meal

Purpose: To radically enhance the digestion and assimilation of food while reducing the body's need to produce digestive enzymes; the higher potency formula will average about three times the potency of the average digestive formula; an average formula may be substituted if three times the regular dose is taken

Each serving should contain approximately:

Amylase blend	22,000 DU	Alpha-galactosidase	450 GALU
Protease blend	80,000 HUT	Phytase	50 PU
Lipase blend	3,000 FCCFIP	Pectinase	50 AJDU
Cellulase blend	2,000 CU	Xylanase	500 XU
Invertase	80 IAU	Hemicellulase	30 HCU
Lactase	900 LacU	Beta-glucanase	25 BGU
Maltase	200 DP	L. acidophilus	250 million CFU
Glucoamylase	50 AGU		

*Probiotic Formula before bed daily

Purpose: To assist the body in balancing microflora

Each serving should contain approximately 5 billion probiotic live cells (guaranteed potency), comprised of:

Bacillus Subtillis	No less than 3 billion CFU guaranteed potency	A blend of L. acidophilus, L. casei, L. bulgaris, L. plantarum, L. rhamnosus, L. salivarius	No less than 1 billion CFU guaranteed potency
L. paracassei F-19	No less than 1 billion CFU guaranteed potency		

*High Cellulase Formula three times daily between meals for one week

Purpose: To manage yeast overgrowth

Each capsule should contain approximately:

Cellulase blend	30,000 CU
Protease blend	100,000 HUT

Contraindications: High amounts of cellulase should not be taken with certain timed-release medications that contain cellulose.

Optional: pH Balancing Formula two times daily

Purpose: To help the body achieve an optimal pH
  Each serving should contain approximately:

Amylase blend	25,000 DU	Lipase blend	175 FCCFIP
Cellulase blend	6,000 CU	Pectinase/Phytase	200 PU
Mineral blend	Potassium bicarbonate, sodium bicarbonate, magnesium citrate	Herbal blend	Hydrilla, marshmallow, papaya
Protease blend	1,000 HUT		

The formula should not exceed 8.0 on the pH scale and the capsule should be enteric coated.

CRAMPS (MUSCLE)

Muscle cramps (painful, involuntary muscle contractions) are generally caused by calcium and magnesium imbalance and/or a vitamin E deficiency. They can also be caused by poor circulation and dehydration. Most muscle cramps that aren't brought on by specific physical activity occur at night, affecting primarily the calf muscles in the legs.

Recommendations include maintaining a well-balanced diet supplemented with vitamins and minerals, maintaining hydration, massage and heat to relieve discomfort, and in cases of frequent cramping, a physical evaluation to rule out impaired circulation. Enzymes can reduce inflammation that may be associated with the cramping, enhance the absorption and digestion of nutrients, and balance the pH in the body.

ENZYME SUPPLEMENTATION SUGGESTIONS:

*pH Balancing Formula two times daily

Purpose: To help the body achieve an optimal pH
  Each serving should contain approximately:

Amylase blend	25,000 DU	Lipase blend	175 FCCFIP
Cellulase blend	6,000 CU	Pectinase/Phytase	200 PU
Mineral blend	Potassium bicarbonate, sodium bicarbonate, magnesium citrate	Herbal blend	Hydrilla, marshmallow, papaya
Protease blend	1,000 HUT		

The formula should not exceed 8.0 on the pH scale and the capsule should be enteric coated.

High Potency Digestive Formula with every meal

Purpose: To radically enhance the digestion and assimilation of food while reducing the body's need to produce digestive enzymes; the higher potency formula will average about three times the potency of the average digestive formula; an average formula may be substituted if three times the regular dose is taken

Each serving should contain approximately:

Amylase blend	22,000 DU	Alpha-galactosidase	450 GALU
Protease blend	80,000 HUT	Phytase	50 PU
Lipase blend	3,000 FCCFIP	Pectinase	50 AJDU
Cellulase blend	2,000 CU	Xylanase	500 XU
Invertase	80 IAU	Hemicellulase	30 HCU
Lactase	900 LacU	Beta-glucanase	25 BGU
Maltase	200 DP	*L. acidophilus*	250 million CFU
Glucoamylase	50 AGU		

Anti-inflammatory Formula at any time for pain relief

Purpose: To address inflammation, speed recovery, and repair tissue; best if enteric coated

Each serving should contain approximately:

Protease blend	120,000 HUT	Amylase blend	7,000 DU
Papain	140,000 PU	Lipase blend	600 FCCFIP
Bromelain	1,200 GDU (11.25 million FCCPU)	Catalase	100 baker units

CROHN'S DISEASE

See INFLAMMATORY BOWEL DISEASE

CYSTIC FIBROSIS

Cystic fibrosis (CF) is a congenital metabolic disorder in which secretions of the exocrine glands (which produce mucus, tears, sweat, saliva, and digestive juices) are abnormal, affecting the respiratory, digestive, and reproductive systems. Excessively viscid mucus obstructs the body's passageways (including pancreatic and bile ducts, intestines, and bronchi), and the sodium and chloride content of sweat increases throughout the patient's life. Symptoms usually appear in childhood and include meconium ileus, poor growth despite good appetite, malabsorption, foul bulky stools, chronic bronchitis with cough, recurrent pneumonia, bronchiectasis, emphysema, clubbing of the fingers, and salt depletion in hot weather.

There are approximately thirty thousand people in the United States with CF, three thousand in Canada, and thirty thousand in other areas of the world. In the United States, there are approximately twenty-five hundred new cases diagnosed each year. Currently, there is no cure for CF.

Enzyme therapy can be used to improve digestion and absorption of nutrients, support the immune system, and reduce the excess mucus being produced by the body.

ENZYME SUPPLEMENTATION SUGGESTIONS:

*High Potency Digestive Formula with every meal

Purpose: To radically enhance the digestion and assimilation of food while reducing the body's need to produce digestive enzymes; the higher potency formula will average about three times the potency of the average digestive formula; an average formula may be substituted if three times the regular dose is taken

Each serving should contain approximately:

Amylase blend	22,000 DU	Alpha-galactosidase	450 GALU
Protease blend	80,000 HUT	Phytase	50 PU
Lipase blend	3,000 FCCFIP	Pectinase	50 AJDU
Cellulase blend	2,000 CU	Xylanase	500 XU
Invertase	80 IAU	Hemicellulase	30 HCU
Lactase	900 LacU	Beta-glucanase	25 BGU
Maltase	200 DP	L. acidophilus	250 million CFU
Glucoamylase	50 AGU		

*Mucolase Formula daily

Purpose: To reduce excess mucus produced by the body; particularly helpful in treating sinus and chest congestion

Each serving should contain approximately:

Mucolase	30 mg

Supporting enzymes:

Amylase blend	7,000 DU	Cellulase blend	200 CU
Protease blend	20,000 HUT	Xylanase	250 XU
Glucoamylase	25 AGU	Pectinase with Phytase	175 endo-PG
Beta-glucanase	30 BGU	Hemicellulase	30 HCU
Lipase blend	250 FCCFIP	Invertase	5 INVU
Alpha-galactosidase	50 GALU		

High Protease Formula three times daily between meals

Purpose: To help support immune function and assist in removing viruses, fungal forms, toxins, bacteria, and heavy metals
Each capsule should contain approximately:

Protease blend	150,000 HUT	Serratiopeptidase	25,000 units
Mucolase	8 mg	Nattokinase blend	400 FU
Catalase	50 baker units		

DANDRUFF

This chronic scalp disorder is the result of dysfunctional sebaceous glands in the scalp, which cause the formation of patches of scaly skin that may burn and itch. Dandruff can be caused by many factors, including poor diet and a mineral, nutrient, or fatty acid deficiency. It can also be a symptom of candidiasis. It is important to recognize the difference between true dandruff and a buildup of hair products, however. Although dandruff is not contagious and is rarely a serious ailment, it can be embarrassing and surprisingly persistent.

Enzymes can be used to improve the functioning of the sebaceous glands by improving the body's ability to digest fats, improve nutrient absorption, reduce excess yeast in the body, and improve the health of the skin.

ENZYME SUPPLEMENTATION SUGGESTIONS:

*High Potency Digestive Formula with every meal

Purpose: To radically enhance the digestion and assimilation of food while reducing the body's need to produce digestive enzymes; the higher potency formula will average about three times the potency of the average digestive formula; an average formula may be substituted if three times the regular dose is taken
Each serving should contain approximately:

Amylase blend	22,000 DU	Alpha-galactosidase	450 GALU
Protease blend	80,000 HUT	Phytase	50 PU
Lipase blend	3,000 FCCFIP	Pectinase	50 AJDU
Cellulase blend	2,000 CU	Xylanase	500 XU
Invertase	80 IAU	Hemicellulase	30 HCU
Lactase	900 LacU	Beta-glucanase	25 BGU
Maltase	200 DP	L. acidophilus	250 million CFU
Glucoamylase	50 AGU		

*High Lipase Formula three times daily between meals with essential fats such as flax oil or fish oil supplements.

Purpose: To improve fat digestion and metabolism, as well as the health of the cardio-vascular system
Each capsule should contain approximately:

Lipase blend	5,000 FCCFIP	Protease blend	20,000 HUT
Amylase blend	10,000 DU	Lactase	300 LacU

High Cellulase Formula three times daily between meals for one week

Purpose: To manage yeast overgrowth
Each capsule should contain approximately:

Cellulase blend	30,000 CU
Protease blend	100,000 HUT

Contraindications: High amounts of cellulase should not be taken with certain timed-release medications that contain cellulose.

High Protease Formula three times daily between meals

Purpose: To help support immune function and assist in removing viruses, fungal forms, toxins, bacteria, and heavy metals
Each capsule should contain approximately:

Protease blend	150,000 HUT	Serratiopeptidase	25,000 units
Mucolase	8 mg	Nattokinase blend	400 FU
Catalase	50 baker units		

DECUBITUS ULCERS

See SKIN ULCERS.

DEPRESSION

Clinical depression may manifest a wide range of symptoms, but the most common are insomnia or hypersomnia, physical hyperactivity or inactivity, feelings of worthlessness, loss of interest or pleasure in usual activities, lack of energy, irritability, either poor appetite and weight loss or increased appetite and weight gain, a diminished ability to think or concentrate, and recurrent thoughts of death or suicide.

Depression may be caused by stress, nutritional deficiencies, allergies, thyroid disorders, sugar, a battle with a serious physical disorder, or chronic fatigue syndrome. Some people also become more depressed in the winter months when there is less exposure to sunlight. It is estimated that seven million Americans suffer from depression each year and more than eight million Americans take antidepressant drugs.

Recommendations include determining what factor(s) are contributing to the depression, eliminating allergens, adding regular physical exercise to a daily routine, and seeking psychological support or counseling. Enzyme therapy can be used to improve nutrient absorption (particularly when eating habits are poor), improve energy levels, mitigate the effects of allergens, and balance the pH and support the immune system in the body to increase overall well-being.

ENZYME SUPPLEMENTATION SUGGESTIONS:

*High Potency Digestive Formula or High Amylase Formula with every meal

Purpose: To radically enhance the digestion and assimilation of food while reducing the body's need to produce digestive enzymes; the higher potency formula will average about three times the potency of the average digestive formula; an average formula may be substituted if three times the regular dose is taken

Each serving should contain approximately:

Amylase blend	22,000 DU	Alpha-galactosidase	450 GALU
Protease blend	80,000 HUT	Phytase	50 PU
Lipase blend	3,000 FCCFIP	Pectinase	50 AJDU
Cellulase blend	2,000 CU	Xylanase	500 XU
Invertase	80 IAU	Hemicellulase	30 HCU
Lactase	900 LacU	Beta-glucanase	25 BGU
Maltase	200 DP	*L. acidophilus*	250 million CFU
Glucoamylase	50 AGU		

*High Protease Formula two times daily between meals

Purpose: To help support immune function and assist in removing viruses, fungal forms, toxins, bacteria, and heavy metals

Each capsule should contain approximately:

Protease blend	150,000 HUT	Serratiopeptidase	25,000 units
Mucolase	8 mg	Nattokinase blend	400 FU
Catalase	50 baker units		

High Amylase Formula at any time to increase energy levels

Purpose: To overcome symptoms of allergies and for the proper digestion of carbohydrates, especially grains, raw vegetables, and legumes
Each serving should contain approximately:

Amylase blend	22,000 DU	Cellulase blend	400 CU
Glucoamylase	30 AGU	Lactase	300 LacU
Alpha-galactosidase	1,000 GALU	Maltase	300 DP
Protease blend	15,000 HUT	Pectinase	20 endo-PG
Lipase blend	150 FCCFIP		

Optional: pH Balancing Formula two times daily

Purpose: To help the body achieve an optimal pH
Each serving should contain approximately:

Amylase blend	25,000 DU	Lipase blend	175 FCCFIP
Cellulase blend	6,000 CU	Pectinase/Phytase	200 PU
Mineral blend	Potassium bicarbonate, sodium bicarbonate, magnesium citrate	Herbal blend	Hydrilla, marshmallow, papaya
Protease blend	1,000 HUT		

The formula should not exceed 8.0 on the pH scale and the capsule should be enteric coated.

DERMATITIS

Also known as eczema, dermatitis is an inflammation of the skin that can result in a rash that is red, itchy, and weepy or patches of skin that are itchy, flaky, scaly, discolored, and thickened. There are three common types of dermatitis: Atopic dermatitis is a chronic form that is often tied to allergies to food or airborne substances. The symptoms are typically an itchy rash in areas of heat or moisture (under the arms, in the groin, behind the knees), skin that is inflamed and accompanied by blisters and scaling, or thickened skin as a result of chronic scratching. Many different environmental factors can aggravate atopic dermatitis. Contact dermatitis is a reaction to an allergen (something the immune system recognizes as foreign) that the skin has come into contact with. Causes may include cosmetics, perfumes, latex or rubber, metal alloys (including silver, nickel, and gold), and poisonous plants, such as poison ivy or poison oak. Contact dermatitis can be cleared up by avoiding exposure to the allergen. Seborrheic dermatitis is a malfunction of the seborrheic glands and can result in scaling of the skin. Dandruff is a form of this condition, as is cradle cap in infants.

Recommendations include treating the body for possible yeast overgrowth and using enzymes to support the digestive and immune systems, detoxify the body, reduce inflammation, and improve circulation to the affected areas to promote healing.

ENZYME SUPPLEMENTATION SUGGESTIONS:

*High Potency Digestive Formula with every meal

Purpose: To radically enhance the digestion and assimilation of food while reducing the body's need to produce digestive enzymes; the higher potency formula will average about three times the potency of the average digestive formula; an average formula may be substituted if three times the regular dose is taken
    Each serving should contain approximately:

Amylase blend	22,000 DU	Alpha-galactosidase	450 GALU
Protease blend	80,000 HUT	Phytase	50 PU
Lipase blend	3,000 FCCFIP	Pectinase	50 AJDU
Cellulase blend	2,000 CU	Xylanase	500 XU
Invertase	80 IAU	Hemicellulase	30 HCU
Lactase	900 LacU	Beta-glucanase	25 BGU
Maltase	200 DP	L. acidophilus	250 million CFU
Glucoamylase	50 AGU		

*High Lipase Formula three times daily between meals with essential fats such as flax oil or fish oil

Purpose: To improve fat digestion and metabolism, as well as the health of the cardiovascular system
    Each capsule should contain approximately:

Lipase blend	5,000 FCCFIP	Protease blend	20,000 HUT
Amylase blend	10,000 DU	Lactase	300 LacU

*Probiotic Formula daily

Purpose: To assist the body in balancing microflora

Each serving should contain approximately 5 billion probiotic live cells (guaranteed potency), comprised of:

Bacillus Subtillis	No less than 3 billion CFU guaranteed potency	A blend of *L. acidophilus, L. casei, L. bulgaris, L. plantarum, L. rhamnosus, L. salivarius*	No less than 1 billion CFU guaranteed potency
L. paracassei F-19	No less than 1 billion CFU guaranteed potency		

High Protease Formula three times daily between meals

Purpose: To help support immune function and assist in removing viruses, fungal forms, toxins, bacteria, and heavy metals
Each capsule should contain approximately:

Protease blend	150,000 HUT	Serratiopeptidase	25,000 units
Mucolase	8 mg	Nattokinase blend	400 FU
Catalase	50 baker units		

Optional: High Amylase Formula three times daily between meals

Purpose: To overcome symptoms of allergies and for the proper digestion of carbohydrates, especially grains, raw vegetables, and legumes
Each serving should contain approximately:

Amylase blend	22,000 DU	Cellulase blend	400 CU
Glucoamylase	30 AGU	Lactase	300 LacU
Alpha-galactosidase	1,000 GALU	Maltase	300 DP
Protease blend	15,000 HUT	Pectinase	20 endo-PG
Lipase blend	150 FCCFIP		

DIABETES

The chronic disorder of diabetes (diabetes mellitus) is a condition characterized by elevated fasting blood glucose levels. This occurs because of an inability to either produce or properly use insulin, a hormone produced by the pancreas that facilitates the absorption of glucose by cells in the tissues of the body. This results in high levels of glucose in the blood and low levels of glucose absorbed by the tissues. Another, very rare type of diabetes is diabetes insipidus, which is a metabolic condition caused by a deficiency of the pituitary hormone. The symptoms are intense thirst and the excretion of large amounts of urine.

There are two types of diabetes mellitus: type 1 and type 2. Type 1 is insulin-dependent diabetes mellitus, which occurs primarily in children and young adults. Type 2 is referred to as adult onset diabetes, because it generally occurs later in life in those with a family history of diabetes. Ninety percent of diabetics are type 2. Contributing factors to the development of this disorder include obesity, genetic predisposition, environmental conditions, nutritional deficiencies, viral infections, and certain chemical exposures that create autoimmunity. In the long-term, diabetics have a greater risk of developing heart disease, of developing kidney disease, of strokes, and of loss of nerve function. Circulation can become a severe problem, leading to various problems in the feet and legs, including a greater risk of gangrene as a result of a foot injury.

Recommendations include management by a physician to maintain normal glucose levels. Vitamins, minerals, and supplementation with animal enzymes from glandular sources (even actual pancreas tissue) may help prevent complications. Enzyme therapy can improve the body's ability to digest and absorb glucose, improve circulation, maintain normal absorption of fats, and balance the body's pH levels.

IMPORTANT NOTE: *Under no circumstances should an individual with diabetes be suddenly taken off of insulin or diabetic drugs. Any nutritional supplementation should be administered only under the close guidance and recommendation of the primary physician.*

ENZYME SUPPLEMENTATION SUGGESTIONS:

*Digestive Formula with every meal

Purpose: To enhance the digestion and assimilation of food while reducing the body's need to produce digestive enzymes

Each serving should contain approximately:
Necessary Ingredients:

Amylase blend	12,000 DU	Alpha-galactosidase	75 GALU
Protease blend	42,000 HUT	Lipase blend	500 FCCFIP
Invertase	10 IAU	Lactase	850 LacU
Maltase	200 DP	Phytase	50 PU
Cellulase blend	200 CU	Pectinase	50 AJDU

Helpful Ingredients:

Xylanase	L. acidophilus
Beta-glucanase	L. bifidus
Hemicellulase	

*High Lipase Formula three times a day on an empty stomach

Purpose: To improve fat digestion and metabolism, as well as the health of the cardio-vascular system
      Each capsule should contain approximately:

Lipase blend	5,000 FCCFIP	Protease blend	20,000 HUT
Amylase blend	10,000 DU	Lactase	300 LacU

High Protease Formula two times per day between meals

Purpose: To help support immune function and assist in removing viruses, fungal forms, toxins, bacteria, and heavy metals
      Each capsule should contain approximately:

Protease blend	150,000 HUT	Serratiopeptidase	25,000 units
Mucolase	8 mg	Nattokinase blend	400 FU
Catalase	50 baker units		

pH Balancing Formula two times per day between meals

Purpose: To help the body achieve an optimal pH
      Each serving should contain approximately:

Amylase blend	25,000 DU	Lipase blend	175 FCCFIP
Cellulase blend	6,000 CU	Pectinase/Phytase	200 PU
Mineral blend	Potassium bicarbonate, sodium bicarbonate, magnesium citrate	Herbal blend	Hydrilla, marshmallow, papaya
Protease blend	1,000 HUT		

      The formula should not exceed 8.0 on the pH scale and the capsule should be enteric coated.

DIARRHEA

Diarrhea is characterized by increased fluidity, frequency (more than four times a day), or volume of bowel movements, as compared to a person's normal pattern of excretion. The causes of diarrhea vary and can include ingestion of certain foods or substances (such as caffeine, artificial sweeteners, or food allergens), food poisoning, viral or bacterial infection, parasites, excessive use of laxatives or antacids, overgrowth of natural bacteria in the intestines, exposure to chemicals the body cannot tolerate, and various bowel disorders or diseases. Acute diarrhea affects almost everyone from time to time. Chronic diarrhea or presence of blood in the stool may be due to a serious intestinal disorder and a physician should be consulted.

Recommendations for treating diarrhea include increased water intake and replacement of electrolytes, probiotic supplements to recolonize and balance friendly intestinal microflora, and avoiding dairy products and solid foods. Enzymes can be used to improve digestion to ensure absorption of nutrients and soothe the gastrointestinal tract.

See IRRITABLE BOWEL SYNDROME and INFLAMMATORY BOWEL DISEASE.

ENZYME SUPPLEMENTATION SUGGESTIONS:

*Digestive Formula with food

Purpose: To enhance the digestion and assimilation of food while reducing the body's need to produce digestive enzymes

Each serving should contain approximately:

Necessary Ingredients:

Amylase blend	12,000 DU	Alpha-galactosidase	75 GALU
Protease blend	42,000 HUT	Lipase blend	500 FCCFIP
Invertase	10 IAU	Lactase	850 LacU
Maltase	200 DP	Phytase	50 PU
Cellulase blend	200 CU	Pectinase	50 AJDU

Helpful Ingredients:

Xylanase	L. acidophilus
Beta-glucanase	L. bifidus
Hemicellulase	

*Soothing Digestive Formula after each episode

Purpose: To help alleviate conditions associated with gastrointestinal distress

Each serving should contain approximately:

Amylase blend	2,000 DU	Gotu kola	50 mg
Lipase blend	175 FCCFIP	Papaya leaf	100 mg
Cellulase blend	400 CU	Prickly ash bark	50 mg
Marshmallow root	100 mg		

Additional helpful ingredients:

DGL (deglycyrrhizinated licorice)	

This formula should *not* contain protease. Other herbs may also be present.

*Probiotic Formula three times a day until symptoms subside, then once daily

Purpose: To assist the body in balancing microflora

Each serving should contain approximately 5 billion probiotic live cells (guaranteed potency), comprised of:

Bacillus Subtillis	No less than 3 billion CFU guaranteed potency	A blend of *L. acidophilus, L. casei, L. bulgaris, L. plantarum, L. rhamnosus, L. salivarius*	No less than 1 billion CFU guaranteed potency
L. paracassei F-19	No less than 1 billion CFU guaranteed potency		

DIVERTICULOSIS/DIVERTICULITIS

Diverticulosis is a condition in which small sacs or pouches (called diverticula) branch out from the large intestine. This occurs when the inner mucosal lining of the intestine protrudes through weak spots in the colon wall. Diverticulosis typically develops with age, and is common after age forty. Contributing factors include stress, obesity, poor diet and eating habits, family history, gallbladder disease, and coronary artery disease.

Typically, individuals with diverticulosis do not have physical symptoms, but symptoms can include tenderness on the left side of the abdomen that is relieved by a bowel movement or passage of gas, cramping, nausea, or constipation or diarrhea.

Diverticulitis can develop from diverticulosis. Diverticulitis is a condition in which the diverticula become inflamed, are perforated, or rupture. Tissue surrounding the colon can become infected. The symptoms include abdominal pain and tenderness, cramping, nausea, fever, and constipation or diarrhea.

Recommendations include a well-balanced, high-fiber diet; stress management; increased water intake; regular exercise; probiotic supplements to colonize the gastrointestinal tract; and nutritional support to optimize digestion and absorption of nutrients. Enzymes can support digestive health, support the balance of healthy intestinal flora, reduce inflammation, help maintain normal pH levels, and help avoid constipation or diarrhea.

ENZYME SUPPLEMENTATION SUGGESTIONS:

*High Potency Digestive Formula with every meal

Purpose: To radically enhance the digestion and assimilation of food while reducing the body's need to produce digestive enzymes; the higher potency formula will average about three times the potency of the average digestive formula; an average formula may be substituted if three times the regular dose is taken
    Each serving should contain approximately:

Amylase blend	22,000 DU	Alpha-galactosidase	450 GALU
Protease blend	80,000 HUT	Phytase	50 PU
Lipase blend	3,000 FCCFIP	Pectinase	50 AJDU
Cellulase blend	2,000 CU	Xylanase	500 XU
Invertase	80 IAU	Hemicellulase	30 HCU
Lactase	900 LacU	Beta-glucanase	25 BGU
Maltase	200 DP	L. acidophilus	250 million CFU
Glucoamylase	50 AGU		

*Probiotic Formula daily

Purpose: To assist the body in balancing microflora
    Each serving should contain approximately 5 billion probiotic live cells (guaranteed potency), comprised of:

Bacillus Subtillis	No less than 3 billion CFU guaranteed potency	A blend of L. acidophilus, L. casei, L. bulgaris, L. plantarum, L. rhamnosus, L. salivarius	No less than 1 billion CFU guaranteed potency
L. paracassei F-19	No less than 1 billion CFU guaranteed potency		

*Soothing Digestive Formula for inflammation as needed

Purpose: To help alleviate conditions associated with gastrointestinal distress
    Each serving should contain approximately:

Amylase blend	2,000 DU	Gotu kola	50 mg
Lipase blend	175 FCCFIP	Papaya leaf	100 mg
Cellulase blend	400 CU	Prickly ash bark	50 mg
Marshmallow root	100 mg		

Additional helpful ingredients:

DGL (deglycyrrhizinated licorice)	

This formula should *not* contain protease. Other herbs may also be present.

High Cellulase Formula three times daily between meals for one to two weeks

Purpose: To manage yeast overgrowth
  Each capsule should contain approximately:

Cellulase blend	30,000 CU
Protease blend	100,000 HUT

Contraindications: High amounts of cellulase should not be taken with certain timed-release medications that contain cellulose.

pH Balancing Formula three times daily between meals

Purpose: To help the body achieve an optimal pH
  Each serving should contain approximately:

Amylase blend	25,000 DU	Lipase blend	175 FCCFIP
Cellulase blend	6,000 CU	Pectinase/Phytase	200 PU
Mineral blend	Potassium bicarbonate, sodium bicarbonate, magnesium citrate	Herbal blend	Hydrilla, marshmallow, papaya
Protease blend	1,000 HUT		

The formula should not exceed 8.0 on the pH scale and the capsule should be enteric coated.

DYSPEPSIA

See INDIGESTION.

EAR INFECTION

Infection of the middle (the eardrum and surrounding structure) or outer ear (the external part of the ear and the ear canal) can cause pressure to build up in tiny spaces that can place pressure on delicate nerve endings, causing pain. The most common type of ear infection is swimmer's ear (*external otitis*), usually caused by bacteria in the ear. Water trapped in the ear can make ear infections more likely. Symptoms include discharge from the ear, slight fever, a pain that intensifies when the ear is pulled or touched, and possibly a temporary loss of hearing.

Otitis media or middle ear infections are caused by bacteria or viruses and are most common in infants and young children. Symptoms include a high fever (103° F or higher), earache, and a feeling of fullness or pressure in the ear. Children will often pull at their ears. This infection is usually a result of bacteria or viruses from the back of the throat moving into the middle ear, but it can be triggered by decompression in air travel, increased exposure to cold climates and high altitudes, exposure to smoking or to wood-burning stoves, and a lowered resistance due to an allergy or upper respiratory infection.

Recommendations include a well-balanced diet, ruling out food allergies that can compromise the immune system, and enzyme supplements to improve overall digestion, absorption of nutrients, and the strength of the immune system.

ENZYME SUPPLEMENTATION SUGGESTIONS:

IMPORTANT NOTE: *Use reduced dosages for younger children.*

*High Protease Formula three times daily on an empty stomach

Purpose: To help support immune function and assist in removing viruses, fungal forms, toxins, bacteria, and heavy metals
Each capsule should contain approximately:

Protease blend	150,000 HUT	Serratiopeptidase	25,000 units
Mucolase	8 mg	Nattokinase blend	400 FU
Catalase	50 baker units		

Digestive Formula with every meal

Purpose: To enhance the digestion and assimilation of food while reducing the body's need to produce digestive enzymes
Each serving should contain approximately:
Necessary Ingredients:

Amylase blend	12,000 DU	Alpha-galactosidase	75 GALU
Protease blend	42,000 HUT	Lipase blend	500 FCCFIP
Invertase	10 IAU	Lactase	850 LacU
Maltase	200 DP	Phytase	50 PU
Cellulase blend	200 CU	Pectinase	50 AJDU

Helpful Ingredients:

Xylanase	L. acidophilus
Beta-glucanase	L. bifidus
Hemicellulase	

ECZEMA

See DERMATITIS.

EDEMA (WATER RETENTION)

Water accounts for more than half of our body weight and is exchanged constantly between the blood and tissues. Water is forced out of the capillaries and into the tissues by the pressure of blood being pumped throughout the body. Through a reverse process that depends on the water-drawing power of proteins in the blood, the capillaries leading from the tissues reabsorb water.

This balance is maintained by the action of the kidneys, which pass excess salt from the blood into the urine to be excreted from the body. Edema can be a problem after surgeries, with prolonged bed rest or hospitalization, with pregnancy, and in a variety of other circumstances. Any nutritional remedies depend on determining the underlying cause or imbalance that created this condition, but enzymes can support the balance of the body's systems, improve digestion and circulation, maintain a normal pH, and reduce excess yeast in the body.

ENZYME SUPPLEMENTATION SUGGESTIONS:

*High Protease Formula three times a day on an empty stomach.

Purpose: In addition to helping support immune function and assist in removing viruses, fungal forms, toxins, bacteria, and heavy metals, it also serves as a diuretic
Each capsule should contain approximately:

Protease blend	150,000 HUT	Serratiopeptidase	25,000 units
Mucolase	8 mg	Nattokinase blend	400 FU
Catalase	50 baker units		

*pH Balancing Formula three times daily between meals

Purpose: To help the body achieve an optimal pH
Each serving should contain approximately:

Amylase blend	25,000 DU	Lipase blend	175 FCCFIP
Cellulase blend	6,000 CU	Pectinase/Phytase	200 PU
Mineral blend	Potassium bicarbonate, sodium bicarbonate, magnesium citrate	Herbal blend	Hydrilla, marshmallow, papaya
Protease blend	1,000 HUT		

The formula should not exceed 8.0 on the pH scale and the capsule should be enteric coated.

High Potency Digestive Formula with every meal

Purpose: To radically enhance the digestion and assimilation of food while reducing the body's need to produce digestive enzymes; the higher potency formula will average about three times the potency of the average digestive formula; an average formula may be substituted if three times the regular dose is taken

Each serving should contain approximately:

Amylase blend	22,000 DU	Alpha-galactosidase	450 GALU
Protease blend	80,000 HUT	Phytase	50 PU
Lipase blend	3,000 FCCFIP	Pectinase	50 AJDU
Cellulase blend	2,000 CU	Xylanase	500 XU
Invertase	80 IAU	Hemicellulase	30 HCU
Lactase	900 LacU	Beta-glucanase	25 BGU
Maltase	200 DP	*L. acidophilus*	250 million CFU
Glucoamylase	50 AGU		

ENDOCRINE GLANDS (SUPPORT)

All of the glands in our body require nutritional support and replenishment. Their ongoing work includes production of hormones, maintaining circulation, regulation of metabolic activities and nutrient levels, maintaining pH balance, managing stress, secreting enzymes to aid in digestion, and regulating development of sexual characteristics. When the body becomes compromised in any way, it can become depleted of vital nutrients that sustain the health of the glands. When one gland is not functioning optimally, the health and activities of all of the other glands can also be affected. (See also HYPOTHYROIDISM, DIABETES, PITUITARY IMBALANCES.)

Signs of poor endocrine function are low estrogen or testosterone levels, which can result in a wide variety of symptoms, including lowered sex drive, infertility, fatigue, feeling hot or cold, mood swings, and excessive sweating.

Recommendations for supporting the health of your endocrine system include detoxification (through the process in chapter 4), nutritional therapies, lowering stress levels, and proper rest, as well as enzymes to support the digestive and immune systems and balance the body's pH levels.

ENZYME SUPPLEMENTATION SUGGESTIONS:

*High Potency Digestive Formula with every meal

Purpose: To radically enhance the digestion and assimilation of food while reducing the body's need to produce digestive enzymes; the higher potency formula will average about three times the potency of the average digestive formula; an average formula may be substituted if three times the regular dose is taken

Each serving should contain approximately:

Amylase blend	22,000 DU	Alpha-galactosidase	450 GALU
Protease blend	80,000 HUT	Phytase	50 PU
Lipase blend	3,000 FCCFIP	Pectinase	50 AJDU
Cellulase blend	2,000 CU	Xylanase	500 XU
Invertase	80 IAU	Hemicellulase	30 HCU
Lactase	900 LacU	Beta-glucanase	25 BGU
Maltase	200 DP	L. acidophilus	250 million CFU
Glucoamylase	50 AGU		

*High Lipase Formula three times a day between meals

Purpose: To improve fat digestion and metabolism, as well as the health of the cardiovascular system

Each capsule should contain approximately:

Lipase blend	5,000 FCCFIP	Protease blend	20,000 HUT
Amylase blend	10,000 DU	Lactase	300 LacU

pH Balancing Formula three times daily between meals

Purpose: To help the body achieve an optimal pH

Each serving should contain approximately:

Amylase blend	25,000 DU	Lipase blend	175 FCCFIP
Cellulase blend	6,000 CU	Pectinase/Phytase	200 PU
Mineral blend	Potassium bicarbonate, sodium bicarbonate, magnesium citrate	Herbal blend	Hydrilla, marshmallow, papaya
Protease blend	1,000 HUT		

The formula should not exceed 8.0 on the pH scale and the capsule should be enteric coated.

ENERGY/ENDURANCE

All activities of the body require energy, and all the body's needs are met by the consumption of foods containing energy in a chemical form. Our diet is made up of three main sources of energy: carbohydrates, proteins, and fats. Carbohydrates are the most readily available source of energy to activate muscles. Proteins work to build and restore body tissue. Fats are the most concentrated form of energy. In a healthy body, it is important to maintain a balance of these energy sources. A lack of energy and endurance can be caused by numerous factors, which may include poor diet, stress, malabsorption of nutrients, a lack of enzymes, free radical damage, and hormonal imbalances.

If you have ever wandered through the local health food store's sports supplement or bodybuilding aisle, no doubt you have noticed that there is no shortage of nutritional supplements and powders. All claim to be cutting-edge nutrition for building muscle, reducing fat, decreasing recovery time, or boosting endurance. Though many of these products work as advertised in ideal situations, a real lack of basic nutrition and effective delivery of nutrients is evident in people who rely heavily on these supplements. If the protein powder you're taking is poorly digested, of what real benefit is it?

Nutrients, whether in the form of food or supplements, can only be delivered to the cells by an enzyme or enzymes. Thus, proper digestion and assimilation of nutrients are vital for good health, physical fitness, energy, and endurance. Many people fill their bodies with vitamins, proteins, and specialty supplements that lack the necessary enzymes to deliver these essential nutrients in the proper amounts to the proper places.

The reason large amounts of supplements are often recommended has little to do with the body's need for such high quantities. Rather it has to do with the body's inability to assimilate such supplements. Therefore, to ensure that at least some of the nutrients are delivered, energy-seekers take enormous amounts of specific nutrients.

The solution is simple. Instead of taking megadoses of supplemental nutrients, add a high-quality digestive enzyme to all meals and supplements you consume so that your body can assimilate them properly. This crucial step can make a dramatic improvement for individuals, whether they are working long hours, taking care of three kids, or training for a triathlon. Since most supplements should be taken with food, enzymes taken with meals will help deliver the nutrients in both the meal *and* the supplement.

For supplements that are designed to be taken on an empty stomach, a broad enzyme blend is recommended for optimum delivery. In addition, a new substance called Bioperine, a phytonutrient, has been shown to increase the absorption of specific vitamins and minerals. It has also been shown to stimulate thermogenesis, which is the metabolic process that produces energy at the cellular level, and thereby increase the energy that can be used for nutrient absorption (see chapter 4).

ENZYME SUPPLEMENTATION SUGGESTIONS:

*High Potency Digestive Formula with every meal

Purpose: To radically enhance the digestion and assimilation of food while reducing the body's need to produce digestive enzymes; the higher potency formula will average about three times the potency of the average digestive formula; an average formula may be substituted if three times the regular dose is taken

Each serving should contain approximately:

Amylase blend	22,000 DU	Alpha-galactosidase	450 GALU
Protease blend	80,000 HUT	Phytase	50 PU
Lipase blend	3,000 FCCFIP	Pectinase	50 AJDU
Cellulase blend	2,000 CU	Xylanase	500 XU
Invertase	80 IAU	Hemicellulase	30 HCU
Lactase	900 LacU	Beta-glucanase	25 BGU
Maltase	200 DP	L. acidophilus	250 million CFU
Glucoamylase	50 AGU		

*Anti-inflammatory Enzyme Formula before and after physical activity

Purpose: To address inflammation, speed recovery, and repair tissue; best if enteric coated

Each serving should contain approximately:

Protease blend	120,000 HUT	Amylase blend	7,000 DU
Papain	140,000 PU	Lipase blend	600 FCCFIP
Bromelain	1,200 GDU (11.25 million FCCPU)	Catalase	100 baker units

Nutrient Enhance Formula when taking vitamins or other nutritional supplements

Purpose: To help the body benefit from supplemental vitamins, minerals, and herbs
Each serving should contain approximately:

Bioperine	5 mg	Lactase	150 ALU
Amylase blend	6,000 DU	Beta-glucanase	90 BGU
Protease blend	10,000 HUT	Xylanase	150 XU
Maltase	100 DP	Pectinase	40 PU
Glucoamylase	25 AGU	Hemicellulase	800 HCU
Alpha-galactosidase	250 GALU	Invertase	79 INVU
Lipase blend	400 FCCFIP	L. acidophilus	150 million CFU
Cellulase blend	500 CU		

High Protease Formula three times daily between meals

Purpose: To help support immune function and assist in removing viruses, fungal forms, toxins, bacteria, and heavy metals
Each capsule should contain approximately:

Protease blend	150,000 HUT	Serratiopeptidase	25,000 units
Mucolase	8 mg	Nattokinase blend	400 FU
Catalase	50 baker units		

Optional: High Amylase Formula anytime a boost in energy is needed

Purpose: For the proper digestion of carbohydrates, especially grains, raw vegetables, and legumes
Each serving should contain approximately:

Amylase blend	22,000 DU	Cellulase blend	400 CU
Glucoamylase	30 AGU	Lactase	300 LacU
Alpha-galactosidase	1,000 GALU	Maltase	300 DP
Protease blend	15,000 HUT	Pectinase	20 endo-PG
Lipase blend	150 FCCFIP		

ENVIRONMENTAL TOXICITY

Today's world is filled with an array of chemicals, toxins, radiation, and heavy metals that have contaminated our water, air, and food. When the body is constantly exposed to and threatened by these environmental toxins, the immune system can become depleted. A compromised immune system, in turn, can contribute to the development of imbalances and disease in the body.

Recommendations include hair, urine, and/or blood assays to determine if any specific underlying toxins exist, particularly in cases of known exposure; taking supplemental enzymes, nutrients, and antioxidants to support the digestive and immune systems and balance the body's pH; establishing a healthy diet; stress management; adequate rest; regular physical exercise; and detoxification of the specific toxin(s) through sauna therapy and drainage remedies to expedite the release of those toxins from the body.

ENZYME SUPPLEMENTATION SUGGESTIONS:

*High Potency Digestive Formula with every meal

Purpose: To radically enhance the digestion and assimilation of food while reducing the body's need to produce digestive enzymes; the higher potency formula will average about three times the potency of the average digestive formula; an average formula may be substituted if three times the regular dose is taken

Each serving should contain approximately:

Amylase blend	22,000 DU	Alpha-galactosidase	450 GALU
Protease blend	80,000 HUT	Phytase	50 PU
Lipase blend	3,000 FCCFIP	Pectinase	50 AJDU
Cellulase blend	2,000 CU	Xylanase	500 XU
Invertase	80 IAU	Hemicellulase	30 HCU
Lactase	900 LacU	Beta-glucanase	25 BGU
Maltase	200 DP	L. acidophilus	250 million CFU
Glucoamylase	50 AGU		

*High Protease Formula three times daily between meals

Purpose: To help support immune function and assist in removing viruses, fungal forms, toxins, bacteria, and heavy metals

Each capsule should contain approximately:

Protease blend	150,000 HUT	Serratiopeptidase	25,000 units
Mucolase	8 mg	Nattokinase blend	400 FU
Catalase	50 baker units		

pH Balancing Formula three times daily between meals

Purpose: To help the body achieve an optimal pH

Each serving should contain approximately:

Amylase blend	25,000 DU	Lipase blend	175 FCCFIP
Cellulase blend	6,000 CU	Pectinase/Phytase	200 PU
Mineral blend	Potassium bicarbonate, sodium bicarbonate, magnesium citrate	Herbal blend	Hydrilla, marshmallow, papaya
Protease blend	1,000 HUT		

The formula should not exceed 8.0 on the pH scale and the capsule should be enteric coated.

EPSTEIN-BARR VIRUS

The Epstein-Barr virus is a very common herpes virus that, once contracted, remains dormant in the cells of the body for the rest of a person's life. In the United States, as many as 95 percent of adults between 35 and 40 years of age have been infected at some point in their lives. In many instances, the symptoms are mild and similar to other common viruses. However, in 35 to 50 percent of adults, EBV develops into infectious mononucleosis. In circumstances when the immune system is compromised, EBV can become reactivated repeatedly, compromising and disrupting immunity, which can lead to other disorders such as chronic fatigue syndrome or fibromyalgia.

Recommendations include optimizing and supporting the immune system; viral detoxification with a high protease enzyme formula; establishing a healthy, well-balanced diet; eliminating food allergens that tax the immune system; and getting appropriate sleep and exercise. Enzymes can be used to support the immune system, improve nutrient absorption, and balance the body's pH to maintain overall health. Enzymes can also be used to treat the symptoms of EBV, such as inflammation and lack of energy.

(See also CHRONIC FATIGUE SYNDROME and FIBROMYALGIA.)

ENZYME SUPPLEMENTATION SUGGESTIONS:

*High Potency Digestive Formula with every meal

Purpose: To radically enhance the digestion and assimilation of food while reducing the body's need to produce digestive enzymes; the higher potency formula will average about three times the potency of the average digestive formula; an average formula may be substituted if three times the regular dose is taken

Each serving should contain approximately:

Amylase blend	22,000 DU	Alpha-galactosidase	450 GALU
Protease blend	80,000 HUT	Phytase	50 PU
Lipase blend	3,000 FCCFIP	Pectinase	50 AJDU
Cellulase blend	2,000 CU	Xylanase	500 XU
Invertase	80 IAU	Hemicellulase	30 HCU
Lactase	900 LacU	Beta-glucanase	25 BGU
Maltase	200 DP	L. acidophilus	250 million CFU
Glucoamylase	50 AGU		

*High Protease Formula three times daily

Purpose: To help support immune function and assist in removing viruses, fungal forms, toxins, bacteria, and heavy metals

Each capsule should contain approximately:

Protease blend	150,000 HUT	Serratiopeptidase	25,000 units
Mucolase	8 mg	Nattokinase blend	400 FU
Catalase	50 baker units		

pH Balancing Formula three times daily between meals

Purpose: To help the body achieve an optimal pH

Each serving should contain approximately:

Amylase blend	25,000 DU	Lipase blend	175 FCCFIP
Cellulase blend	6,000 CU	Pectinase/Phytase	200 PU
Mineral blend	Potassium bicarbonate, sodium bicarbonate, magnesium citrate	Herbal blend	Hydrilla, marshmallow, papaya
Protease blend	1,000 HUT		

The formula should not exceed 8.0 on the pH scale and the capsule should be enteric coated.

Optional: Anti-inflammatory Formula may be added for inflammation

Purpose: To address inflammation, speed recovery, and repair tissue; best if enteric coated

Each serving should contain approximately:

Protease blend	120,000 HUT	Amylase blend	7,000 DU
Papain	140,000 PU	Lipase blend	600 FCCFIP
Bromelain	1,200 GDU (11.25 million FCCPU)	Catalase	100 baker units

Optional: High Amylase Formula may be added for increased energy

Purpose: To overcome symptoms of allergies and for the proper digestion of carbohydrates, especially grains, raw vegetables, and legumes

Each serving should contain approximately:

Amylase blend	22,000 DU	Cellulase blend	400 CU
Glucoamylase	30 AGU	Lactase	300 LacU
Alpha-galactosidase	1,000 GALU	Maltase	300 DP
Protease blend	15,000 HUT	Pectinase	20 endo-PG
Lipase blend	150 FCCFIP		

ERECTILE DYSFUNCTION

Erectile dysfunction is a form of sexual dysfunction characterized by the inability to develop or maintain an erection of the penis for satisfactory sexual intercourse, regardless of the capacity for ejaculation. This condition currently affects ten to twenty million American men, and 5 percent of men over the age of fifty.

Causes of impotence can include vascular insufficiency, stress, certain drugs, neurological diseases, endocrine disorders (including diabetes and hypothyroidism), certain diseases of or trauma to the male sexual organs, excessive use of alcohol and tobacco products, and psychological factors.

Recommendations include a healthy, well-balanced diet high in quality protein, regular exercise, increasing vitamin and mineral intake, and avoiding smoking and alcohol. Enzymes can be used to improve circulation, improve hormonal balances, and support overall health by aiding digestion.

ENZYME SUPPLEMENTATION SUGGESTIONS:

*High Potency Digestive Formula with every meal

Purpose: To radically enhance the digestion and assimilation of food while reducing the body's need to produce digestive enzymes; the higher potency formula will average about three times the potency of the average digestive formula; an average formula may be substituted if three times the regular dose is taken

Each serving should contain approximately:

Amylase blend	22,000 DU	Alpha-galactosidase	450 GALU
Protease blend	80,000 HUT	Phytase	50 PU
Lipase blend	3,000 FCCFIP	Pectinase	50 AJDU
Cellulase blend	2,000 CU	Xylanase	500 XU
Invertase	80 IAU	Hemicellulase	30 HCU
Lactase	900 LacU	Beta-glucanase	25 BGU
Maltase	200 DP	L. acidophilus	250 million CFU
Glucoamylase	50 AGU		

*Nattokinase Formula three times daily morning and night (for circulation)

Purpose: To support cardiovascular health and decrease blood pressure by breaking down fibrin

Each serving should contain approximately:
Necessary ingredient:

Nattokinase NSK-SD	1,000 FU

Helpful ingredients:

Amylase blend	9,000 DU	Glucoamylase	25 AGU
Protease blend	20,000 HUT	Lipase blend	1,000 FCCFIP
Minerals	85 mg	Cellulase blend	400 CU

High Lipase Formula three times daily morning and night (for hormones)

Purpose: To improve fat digestion and metabolism, as well as the health of the cardiovascular system

Each capsule should contain approximately:

Lipase blend	5,000 FCCFIP	Protease blend	20,000 HUT
Amylase blend	10,000 DU	Lactase	300 LacU

EXERCISE

Exercise is defined as physical exertion to improve health. It should be a vital and significant part of everyone's life. Talk to your physician about how much exercise is right for you. A reasonable goal for many people is to work up to exercising four to six times a week for thirty to sixty minutes at a time. Remember, though, that exercise has so many benefits that any amount is better than none. Start out slowly. If you've been inactive for years, you can't run the Boston Marathon after two weeks of training. Begin with a ten-minute period of light exercise, or a brisk walk every day. Then gradually increase how hard you exercise and for how long.

The benefits of regular exercise include reducing your risk of heart disease, high blood pressure, osteoporosis, diabetes, and obesity; keeping joints, tendons, and ligaments flexible; improved mental well-being; relief of stress and anxiety; and maintenance of normal weight through increased metabolism. Enzymes can be used to support a healthy exercise regimen by improving nutrient absorption in order to increase energy levels and endurance, reducing inflammation that may occur as a result of exercise, improving circulation to help tissues repair after exercise, and balancing the body's pH, which can suffer as a result of lactic acid buildup in the muscles.

See also ATHLETIC PERFORMANCE and ENERGY AND ENDURANCE.

ENZYME SUPPLEMENTATION SUGGESTIONS:

*High Potency Digestive Formula with every meal

Purpose: To radically enhance the digestion and assimilation of food while reducing the body's need to produce digestive enzymes; the higher potency formula will average about three times the potency of the average digestive formula; an average formula may be substituted if three times the regular dose is taken

Each serving should contain approximately:

Amylase blend	22,000 DU	Alpha-galactosidase	450 GALU
Protease blend	80,000 HUT	Phytase	50 PU
Lipase blend	3,000 FCCFIP	Pectinase	50 AJDU
Cellulase blend	2,000 CU	Xylanase	500 XU
Invertase	80 IAU	Hemicellulase	30 HCU
Lactase	900 LacU	Beta-glucanase	25 BGU
Maltase	200 DP	L. acidophilus	250 million CFU
Glucoamylase	50 AGU		

*Anti-inflammatory Formula before and after physical activity

Purpose: To address inflammation, speed recovery, and repair tissue; best if enteric coated

Each serving should contain approximately:

Protease blend	120,000 HUT	Amylase blend	7,000 DU
Papain	140,000 PU	Lipase blend	600 FCCFIP
Bromelain	1,200 GDU (11.25 million FCCPU)	Catalase	100 baker units

*Nutrient Enhance Formula when taking vitamins, minerals or herbs.

Purpose: To help the body benefit from supplemental vitamins, minerals, and herbs

Each serving should contain approximately:

Bioperine	5 mg	Lactase	150 ALU
Amylase blend	6,000 DU	Beta-glucanase	90 BGU
Protease blend	10,000 HUT	Xylanase	150 XU
Maltase	100 DP	Pectinase	40 PU
Glucoamylase	25 AGU	Hemicellulase	800 HCU
Alpha-galactosidase	250 GALU	Invertase	79 INVU
Lipase blend	400 FCCFIP	L. acidophilus	150 million CFU
Cellulase blend	500 CU		

*pH Balancing Formula two times per day morning and night

Purpose: To help the body achieve an optimal pH

Each serving should contain approximately:

Amylase blend	25,000 DU	Lipase blend	175 FCCFIP
Cellulase blend	6,000 CU	Pectinase/Phytase	200 PU
Mineral blend	Potassium bicarbonate, sodium bicarbonate, magnesium citrate	Herbal blend	Hydrilla, marshmallow, papaya
Protease blend	1,000 HUT		

The formula should not exceed 8.0 on the pH scale and the capsule should be enteric coated.

Optional: High Protease Formula two times per day morning and night

Purpose: To help support immune function and assist in removing viruses, fungal forms, toxins, bacteria, and heavy metals

Each capsule should contain approximately:

Protease blend	150,000 HUT	Serratiopeptidase	25,000 units
Mucolase	8 mg	Nattokinase blend	400 FU
Catalase	50 baker units		

Optional: Serratiopeptidase Formula may be added before and after physical activity for great benefit

Purpose: To break down protein and reduce inflammation. Also supports cardiovascular health and enhances other proteases.

Each serving should contain approximately:

Serratiopeptidase	80,000 SU
Protease blend	70,000 HUT
Mineral blend	50 mg

EYE CONDITIONS

Like all other parts of the body, the eyes require special nutrients in order to remain healthy. Additionally, the health and appearance of the eyes can also serve as a strong indicator of imbalances in other parts of the body. For example,

- Thyroid imbalances may be indicated by bulging or protruding eyes.

- Allergies may be indicated by swelling, redness, and irritation of the eyes, and/or dark circles under the eyes.

- Colds may be indicated by watery eyes.

- Liver or gallbladder disease may be indicated by yellowing eyes.

- Diabetes or hypertension may be indicated by periodic blurred vision.

Therapeutic considerations for eye conditions include avoiding eyestrain, eating a well-balanced diet, supplementing the diet with antioxidants to protect against free radical damage, and the addition of enzymes or supplemental nutrients to help maintain health and a viable digestive and immune system.

It is always wise to consult with a physician in cases of infections or serious eye imbalances, such as pinkeye, shingles, ulcerations near the eye, glaucoma, macular degeneration, or detached retinas.

ENZYME SUPPLEMENTATION SUGGESTIONS:

*High Potency Digestive Formula with every meal

Purpose: To radically enhance the digestion and assimilation of food while reducing the body's need to produce digestive enzymes; the higher potency formula will average about three times the potency of the average digestive formula; an average formula may be substituted if three times the regular dose is taken

Each serving should contain approximately:

Amylase blend	22,000 DU	Alpha-galactosidase	450 GALU
Protease blend	80,000 HUT	Phytase	50 PU
Lipase blend	3,000 FCCFIP	Pectinase	50 AJDU
Cellulase blend	2,000 CU	Xylanase	500 XU
Invertase	80 IAU	Hemicellulase	30 HCU
Lactase	900 LacU	Beta-glucanase	25 BGU
Maltase	200 DP	*L. acidophilus*	250 million CFU
Glucoamylase	50 AGU		

*High Protease Formula three times daily to increase circulation

Purpose: To help support immune function and assist in removing viruses, fungal forms, toxins, bacteria, and heavy metals

Each capsule should contain approximately:

Protease blend	150,000 HUT	Serratiopeptidase	25,000 units
Mucolase	8 mg	Nattokinase blend	400 FU
Catalase	50 baker units		

*Nattokinase Formula three times daily to increase circulation

Purpose: To support cardiovascular health and decrease blood pressure by breaking down fibrin

Each serving should contain approximately:
Necessary ingredient:

Nattokinase NSK-SD	1,000 FU

Helpful ingredients:

Amylase blend	9,000 DU	Glucoamylase	25 AGU
Protease blend	20,000 HUT	Lipase blend	1,000 FCCFIP
Minerals	85 mg	Cellulase blend	400 CU

FATIGUE

Fatigue is a common complaint that can be associated with overwork, lack of sleep, or poor nutrition. Persistent fatigue may be a result of or result in depression, lowered immune system response, headaches, inflamed throat and lungs, fevers, and swollen lymph glands.

Recommendations include eating a well-balanced diet, allowing time for adequate rest and sleep, managing stress, ascertaining the underlying cause of the fatigue, and supporting the digestive and immune systems with nutritional supplementation and enzymes. For the overall health of the body, these suggestions cannot be emphasized enough. In addition, enzymes can be used to reduce inflammation that may occur as a result of fatigue, maintain a balanced pH in the body to improve overall health, and increase energy levels.

See also CHRONIC FATIGUE SYNDROME.

ENZYME SUPPLEMENTATION SUGGESTIONS:

*High Potency Digestive Formula with every meal

Purpose: To radically enhance the digestion and assimilation of food while reducing the body's need to produce digestive enzymes; the higher potency formula will average about three times the potency of the average digestive formula; an average formula may be substituted if three times the regular dose is taken
Each serving should contain approximately:

Amylase blend	22,000 DU	Alpha-galactosidase	450 GALU
Protease blend	80,000 HUT	Phytase	50 PU
Lipase blend	3,000 FCCFIP	Pectinase	50 AJDU
Cellulase blend	2,000 CU	Xylanase	500 XU
Invertase	80 IAU	Hemicellulase	30 HCU
Lactase	900 LacU	Beta-glucanase	25 BGU
Maltase	200 DP	L. acidophilus	250 million CFU
Glucoamylase	50 AGU		

*pH Balancing Formula three times daily

Purpose: To help the body achieve an optimal pH
Each serving should contain approximately:

Amylase blend	25,000 DU	Lipase blend	175 FCCFIP
Cellulase blend	6,000 CU	Pectinase/Phytase	200 PU
Mineral blend	Potassium bicarbonate, sodium bicarbonate, magnesium citrate	Herbal blend	Hydrilla, marshmallow, papaya
Protease blend	1,000 HUT		

The formula should not exceed 8.0 on the pH scale and the capsule should be enteric coated.

*Anti-inflammatory Formula three times daily for inflammation (more may be added)

Purpose: To address inflammation, speed recovery, and repair tissue; best if enteric coated

Each serving should contain approximately:

Protease blend	120,000 HUT	Amylase blend	7,000 DU
Papain	140,000 PU	Lipase blend	600 FCCFIP
Bromelain	1,200 GDU (11.25 million FCCPU)	Catalase	100 baker units

Serratiopeptidase Formula for inflammation

Purpose: To break down protein and reduce inflammation. Also supports cardiovascular health and enhances other proteases.

Each serving should contain approximately:

Serratiopeptidase	80,000 SU
Protease blend	70,000 HUT
Mineral blend	50 mg

Supporting enzymes:

Bromelain	Papain

High Protease Formula three times daily

Purpose: To help support immune function and assist in removing viruses, fungal forms, toxins, bacteria, and heavy metals

Each capsule should contain approximately:

Protease blend	150,000 HUT	Serratiopeptidase	25,000 units
Mucolase	8 mg	Nattokinase blend	400 FU
Catalase	50 baker units		

High Amylase Formula may be added any time to increase energy level

Purpose: To overcome symptoms of allergies and for the proper digestion of carbohydrates, especially grains, raw vegetables, and legumes

Each serving should contain approximately:

Amylase blend	22,000 DU	Cellulase blend	400 CU
Glucoamylase	30 AGU	Lactase	300 LacU
Alpha-galactosidase	1,000 GALU	Maltase	300 DP
Protease blend	15,000 HUT	Pectinase	20 endo-PG
Lipase blend	150 FCCFIP		

Soothing Digestive Formula as needed

Purpose: To help alleviate conditions associated with gastrointestinal distress

Each serving should contain approximately:

Amylase blend	2,000 DU	Gotu kola	50 mg
Lipase blend	175 FCCFIP	Papaya leaf	100 mg
Cellulase blend	400 CU	Prickly ash bark	50 mg
Marshmallow root	100 mg		

Additional helpful ingredients:

DGL (deglycyrrhizinated licorice)	

FEVER

A fever is a rise in body temperature to greater than 100 degrees Fahrenheit. The body maintains stability between 97 degrees and 100 degrees by balancing the heat produced by its metabolism with the heat lost to the environment. The "thermostat" is located in the hypothalamus within the brain. A fever occurs when the body's thermostat resets at a higher temperature, usually in response to an infection.

A fever may be accompanied by other symptoms such as shivering, headache, sweating, thirst, a flushed face, hot skin, and faster than normal breathing. Fever symptoms indicate the presence of an imbalance or disease process. An elevated temperature can be helpful to the body since it serves to destroy foreign microbes, assisting the body's efforts to eliminate toxins or antigens. High fevers may cause delirium, confusion, dehydration, seizures, or even a coma. Consult a physician if a high fever persists.

Recommendations for treating fevers include increased hydration, rest and sleep, avoiding heavy or solid foods until the condition has improved, and supporting the immune system and maintaining the body's normal pH levels.

ENZYME SUPPLEMENTATION SUGGESTIONS:

*High Protease Formula, Anti-inflammatory Formula, or combination of both, three times daily

Purpose: To help support immune function and assist in removing viruses, fungal forms, toxins, bacteria, and heavy metals

Each capsule should contain approximately:

Protease blend	150,000 HUT	Serratiopeptidase	25,000 units
Mucolase	8 mg	Nattokinase blend	400 FU
Catalase	50 baker units		

Purpose: To address inflammation, speed recovery, and repair tissue; best if enteric coated

Each serving should contain approximately:

Protease blend	120,000 HUT	Amylase blend	7,000 DU
Papain	140,000 PU	Lipase blend	600 FCCFIP
Bromelain	1,200 GDU (11.25 million FCCPU)	Catalase	100 baker units

High Potency Digestive Formula with every meal

Purpose: To radically enhance the digestion and assimilation of food while reducing the body's need to produce digestive enzymes; the higher potency formula will average about three times the potency of the average digestive formula; an average formula may be substituted if three times the regular dose is taken

Each serving should contain approximately:

Amylase blend	22,000 DU	Alpha-galactosidase	450 GALU
Protease blend	80,000 HUT	Phytase	50 PU
Lipase blend	3,000 FCCFIP	Pectinase	50 AJDU
Cellulase blend	2,000 CU	Xylanase	500 XU
Invertase	80 IAU	Hemicellulase	30 HCU
Lactase	900 LacU	Beta-glucanase	25 BGU
Maltase	200 DP	L. acidophilus	250 million CFU
Glucoamylase	50 AGU		

Optional: pH Balancing Formula three times daily

Purpose: To help the body achieve an optimal pH
Each serving should contain approximately:

Amylase blend	25,000 DU	Lipase blend	175 FCCFIP
Cellulase blend	6,000 CU	Pectinase/Phytase	200 PU
Mineral blend	Potassium bicarbonate, sodium bicarbonate, magnesium citrate	Herbal blend	Hydrilla, marshmallow, papaya
Protease blend	1,000 HUT		

The formula should not exceed 8.0 on the pH scale and the capsule should be enteric coated.

FIBROMYALGIA

Fibromyalgia disorder is a condition associated with chronic musculoskeletal pain and fatigue that affects about 4 percent of the population. Research indicates that people with fibromyalgia have defects in the neuroregulatory system, which results in abnormal production of neurotransmitters such as seratonin, melatonin, and dopamine, and other chemicals that help control pain, mood, sleep, and the immune system. This is the reason for the wide array of symptoms associated with this condition.

One of the key symptoms of fibromyalgia is an altered sleep pattern with reduced REM sleep and increased non-REM sleep. Other symptoms include six or more typical, reproducible tender points in the body; joint swelling; generalized stiffness or aches of at least three anatomical sites for at least three months; sleep disturbances; generalized fatigue; numbness or tingling; irritable bowel syndrome; chronic headaches; and neurological and psychological complaints. While the severity of symptoms fluctuates from person to person, fibromyalgia may resemble a post-viral state. Fibromyalgia is very similar to chronic fatigue syndrome (CFS); the only difference is that a diagnosis of CFS requires complaints of fatigue, while a diagnosis of fibromyalgia requires musculoskeletal pain.

Enzyme therapy can be used to reduce inflammation, support the body's digestive and immune systems, and balance the pH levels to support overall health.

See also CHRONIC FATIGUE SYNDROME.

ENZYME SUPPLEMENTATION SUGGESTIONS:

*High Potency Digestive Formula with every meal

Purpose: To radically enhance the digestion and assimilation of food while reducing the body's need to produce digestive enzymes; the higher potency formula will average about three times the potency of the average digestive formula; an average formula may be substituted if three times the regular dose is taken

Each serving should contain approximately:

Amylase blend	22,000 DU	Alpha-galactosidase	450 GALU
Protease blend	80,000 HUT	Phytase	50 PU
Lipase blend	3,000 FCCFIP	Pectinase	50 AJDU
Cellulase blend	2,000 CU	Xylanase	500 XU
Invertase	80 IAU	Hemicellulase	30 HCU
Lactase	900 LacU	Beta-glucanase	25 BGU
Maltase	200 DP	L. acidophilus	250 million CFU
Glucoamylase	50 AGU		

*Anti-inflammatory Formula three times daily or anytime for pain

Purpose: To address inflammation, speed recovery, and repair tissue; best if enteric coated

Each serving should contain approximately:

Protease blend	120,000 HUT	Amylase blend	7,000 DU
Papain	140,000 PU	Lipase blend	600 FCCFIP
Bromelain	1,200 GDU (11.25 million FCCPU)	Catalase	100 baker units

High Protease Formula two times daily, morning and night

Purpose: To help support immune function and assist in removing viruses, fungal forms, toxins, bacteria, and heavy metals

Each capsule should contain approximately:

Protease blend	150,000 HUT	Serratiopeptidase	25,000 units
Mucolase	8 mg	Nattokinase blend	400 FU
Catalase	50 baker units		

pH Balancing Formula three times daily

Purpose: To help the body achieve an optimal pH
    Each serving should contain approximately:

Amylase blend	25,000 DU	Lipase blend	175 FCCFIP
Cellulase blend	6,000 CU	Pectinase/Phytase	200 PU
Mineral blend	Potassium bicarbonate, sodium bicarbonate, magnesium citrate	Herbal blend	Hydrilla, marshmallow, papaya
Protease blend	1,000 HUT		

    The formula should not exceed 8.0 on the pH scale and the capsule should be enteric coated.

Optional: Serratiopeptidase Formula may be added to the anti-inflammatory formula for chronic conditions

Purpose: To break down protein and reduce inflammation. Also supports cardiovascular health and enhances other proteases.
    Each serving should contain approximately:

Serratiopeptidase	80,000 SU
Protease blend	70,000 HUT
Mineral blend	50 mg

Supporting enzymes:

Bromelain	Papain

FLATULENCE

Flatulence is the expulsion of intestinal gases formed by fermentation in the gastrointestinal tract as a result of the action between bacteria, carbohydrates, and proteins in undigested foods. It may be accompanied by abdominal discomfort. Large amounts of gases that cause abdominal discomfort are usually due to intestinal sensitivities, although there are a variety of conditions associated with excess gas in the gastrointestinal tract, such as eating too fast, eating foods that tend to produce gas (cabbage, baked beans), food allergies (lactose intolerance, wheat allergies) and enzyme deficiencies. For more information see IRRITABLE BOWEL SYNDROME, ALLERGIES (FOOD), INFLAMMATORY BOWEL DISEASE.

    Enzymes can be used to improve digestion, particularly the digestion of carbohydrates and sugars, which tend to be the primary cause of excessive gas production, and balance the pH of the body to improve overall health.

ENZYME SUPPLEMENTATION SUGGESTIONS:

*High Amylase Formula with every meal (more may be taken if necessary)

Purpose: For the proper digestion of carbohydrates, especially grains, raw vegetables, and legumes
Each serving should contain approximately:

Amylase blend	22,000 DU	Cellulase blend	400 CU
Glucoamylase	30 AGU	Lactase	300 LacU
Alpha-galactosidase	1,000 GALU	Maltase	300 DP
Protease blend	15,000 HUT	Pectinase	20 endo-PG
Lipase blend	150 FCCFIP		

*Probiotic Formula daily

Purpose: To assist the body in balancing microflora
Each serving should contain approximately 5 billion probiotic live cells (guaranteed potency), comprised of:

Bacillus Subtillis	No less than 3 billion CFU guaranteed potency	A blend of L. acidophilus, L. casei, L. bulgaris, L. plantarum, L. rhamnosus, L. salivarius	No less than 1 billion CFU guaranteed potency
L. paracassei F-19	No less than 1 billion CFU guaranteed potency		

pH balancing Formula before bed

Purpose: To help the body achieve an optimal pH
Each serving should contain approximately:

Amylase blend	25,000 DU	Lipase blend	175 FCCFIP
Cellulase blend	6,000 CU	Pectinase/Phytase	200 PU
Mineral blend	Potassium bicarbonate, sodium bicarbonate, magnesium citrate	Herbal blend	Hydrilla, marshmallow, papaya
Protease blend	1,000 HUT		

The formula should not exceed 8.0 on the pH scale and the capsule should be enteric coated.

FLU
See INFLUENZA.

FUNGUS
See CANDIDIASIS, RINGWORM.

GALLBLADDER IMBALANCES
The gallbladder is a small muscular sac that lies under the liver and expels bile through the common bile duct into the duodenum, which is the first and shortest part of the small intestine and is where most chemical digestion takes place. Gallstones and gallbladder inflammation (cholecystitis) are the most common disorders of the gallbladder and may cause a great deal of discomfort, primarily in the upper right abdominal region. These conditions often occur as a result of regularly eating fatty or fried foods. Other symptoms may include nausea, vomiting, and fever. It is important to consult with a physician in cases of cholecystitis, as untreated cases can be life threatening.

Recommendations to improve or maintain the health and functioning of the gallbladder include eating a healthy, well-balanced diet, using a detoxification program for the liver and colon, and using enzyme therapy to support proper fat metabolism.

IMPORTANT NOTE: *If a smaller dose of enzymes than suggested is consumed, it may result in nausea.*

ENZYME SUPPLEMENTATION SUGGESTIONS:
Acute gallbladder imbalance:

*High Potency Digestive Formula with every meal

Purpose: To radically enhance the digestion and assimilation of food while reducing the body's need to produce digestive enzymes; the higher potency formula will average about three times the potency of the average digestive formula; an average formula may be substituted if three times the regular dose is taken
Each serving should contain approximately:

Amylase blend	22,000 DU	Alpha-galactosidase	450 GALU
Protease blend	80,000 HUT	Phytase	50 PU
Lipase blend	3,000 FCCFIP	Pectinase	50 AJDU
Cellulase blend	2,000 CU	Xylanase	500 XU
Invertase	80 IAU	Hemicellulase	30 HCU
Lactase	900 LacU	Beta-glucanase	25 BGU
Maltase	200 DP	L. acidophilus	250 million CFU
Glucoamylase	50 AGU		

*High Lipase Formula between meals

Purpose: To improve fat digestion and metabolism, as well as the health of the cardio-vascular system

Each capsule should contain approximately:

Lipase blend	5,000 FCCFIP	Protease blend	20,000 HUT
Amylase blend	10,000 DU	Lactase	300 LacU

Chronic gallbladder imbalances:

Soothing Digestive Formula whenever nauseous

Purpose: To help alleviate conditions associated with gastrointestinal distress

Each serving should contain approximately:

Amylase blend	2,000 DU	Gotu kola	50 mg
Lipase blend	175 FCCFIP	Papaya leaf	100 mg
Cellulase blend	400 CU	Prickly ash bark	50 mg
Marshmallow root	100 mg		

Additional helpful ingredients:

DGL (deglycyrrhizinated licorice)	

This formula should *not* contain protease. Other herbs may also be present.

GASTRITIS

Gastritis is a medical term for an inflammation of the mucous membrane that lines the stomach. There are different types of gastritis, ranging from severe to more mild forms. Each type is basically associated with a particular cause. For instance, acute stress gastritis is caused by a severe illness or injury; chronic erosive gastritis is caused by irritants introduced to the stomach and is common among alcoholics; and viral, fungal, or bacterial gastritis is caused by a viral, fungal, or bacterial infection. Other causes of gastritis include bile reflux from the intestine and stress. Each type of gastritis may be acute, occurring as a sudden attack, or chronic, developing gradually over a longer period of time.

The symptoms of gastritis common across the various types include indigestion, stomach or abdominal pain, diarrhea, nausea, vomiting, and possibly appetite loss.

Recommendations for treating gastritis include stress reduction, dietary changes, specific treatment for the underlying cause, and enzymes and nutritional support to soothe the stomach and gastrointestinal tract and to enhance digestion and absorption.

ENZYME SUPPLEMENTATION SUGGESTIONS:

*Digestive Formula with every meal

Purpose: To enhance the digestion and assimilation of food while reducing the body's need to produce digestive enzymes
Each serving should contain approximately:
Necessary Ingredients:

Amylase blend	12,000 DU	Alpha-galactosidase	75 GALU
Protease blend	42,000 HUT	Lipase blend	500 FCCFIP
Invertase	10 IAU	Lactase	850 LacU
Maltase	200 DP	Phytase	50 PU
Cellulase blend	200 CU	Pectinase	50 AJDU

Helpful Ingredients:

Xylanase	L. acidophilus
Beta-glucanase	L. bifidus
Hemicellulase	

*Soothing Digestive Formula after every meal

Purpose: To help alleviate conditions associated with gastrointestinal distress
Each serving should contain approximately:

Amylase blend	2,000 DU	Gotu kola	50 mg
Lipase blend	175 FCCFIP	Papaya leaf	100 mg
Cellulase blend	400 CU	Prickly ash bark	50 mg
Marshmallow root	100 mg		

Additional helpful ingredients:

DGL (deglycyrrhizinated licorice)	

This formula should *not* contain protease. Other herbs may also be present.

*Probiotic Formula daily before bed

Purpose: To assist the body in balancing microflora
    Each serving should contain approximately 5 billion probiotic live cells (guaranteed potency), comprised of:

Bacillus Subtillis	No less than 3 billion CFU guaranteed potency	A blend of *L. acidophilus, L. casei, L. bulgaris, L. plantarum, L. rhamnosus, L. salivarius*	No less than 1 billion CFU guaranteed potency
L. paracassei F-19	No less than 1 billion CFU guaranteed potency		

GASTROESOPHAGEAL REFLUX DISEASE

Heartburn is the major symptom of gastoesophageal reflux disease (GERD). Heartburn occurs when acid from the stomach flows up into the esophagus. GERD is caused when the opening between the stomach and the esophagus (lower esophageal sphincter, or LES) weakens or relaxes at the wrong time. (See also INDIGESTION.) The purpose of the LES is to prevent gastric contents from backing up into the esophagus. Normally, the LES creates pressure, closing the lower end of the esophagus, but relaxes after each swallow to allow food into the stomach. Reflux occurs when the pressure within the stomach exceeds LES pressure; it does not occur because there is too much acid in the stomach. It most often occurs as a result of overeating, stress, allergies, eating certain irritative foods, pregnancy, ulcers, or gallbladder problems. (See also HIATAL HERNIA.) When the gastric juices, which are acidic, rise into the esophagus, a painful burning sensation occurs, usually somewhere between the tip of the breastbone and the throat.

Typically, if reflux occurs more than twice a week, a patient is diagnosed with GERD. The most common symptom of GERD is chronic, frequent heartburn, but some with GERD instead experience a dry cough, asthmalike symptoms, or trouble swallowing. GERD can lead to more serious health issues over time, such as scarring and ulcers in the lining of the esophagus.

The traditional medical treatment for GERD is to prescribe antacids. Antacids not only mask the problem, they also can cause long-term digestive difficulties. Antacids are merely Band-Aids and do nothing to correct the problem.

For people with GERD, it is important to make lifestyle changes, such as reducing stress; stopping smoking; losing weight and getting regular exercise; eating smaller, more frequent meals; chewing food thoroughly; and avoiding lying down for three hours after eating. Enzymes should be used to improve digestion and the absorption of nutrients, soothe the digestive tract, and balance the pH in the body, reducing excessive stomach acid if that is a contributing problem.

ENZYME SUPPLEMENTATION SUGGESTIONS:

*High Potency Digestive Formula with meals

Purpose: To radically enhance the digestion and assimilation of food while reducing the body's need to produce digestive enzymes; the higher potency formula will average about three times the potency of the average digestive formula; an average formula may be substituted if three times the regular dose is taken
Each serving should contain approximately:

Amylase blend	22,000 DU	Alpha-galactosidase	450 GALU
Protease blend	80,000 HUT	Phytase	50 PU
Lipase blend	3,000 FCCFIP	Pectinase	50 AJDU
Cellulase blend	2,000 CU	Xylanase	500 XU
Invertase	80 IAU	Hemicellulase	30 HCU
Lactase	900 LacU	Beta-glucanase	25 BGU
Maltase	200 DP	L. acidophilus	250 million CFU
Glucoamylase	50 AGU		

*Soothing Digestive Formula after every meal

Purpose: To help alleviate conditions associated with gastrointestinal distress
Each serving should contain approximately:

Amylase blend	2,000 DU	Gotu kola	50 mg
Lipase blend	175 FCCFIP	Papaya leaf	100 mg
Cellulase blend	400 CU	Prickly ash bark	50 mg
Marshmallow root	100 mg		

Additional helpful ingredients:

DGL (deglycyrrhizinated licorice)	

This formula should *not* contain protease. Other herbs may also be present.

pH Balancing Formula three times daily

Purpose: To help the body achieve an optimal pH
    Each serving should contain approximately:

Amylase blend	25,000 DU	Lipase blend	175 FCCFIP
Cellulase blend	6,000 CU	Pectinase/Phytase	200 PU
Mineral blend	Potassium bicarbonate, sodium bicarbonate, magnesium citrate	Herbal blend	Hydrilla, marshmallow, papaya
Protease blend	1,000 HUT		

The formula should not exceed 8.0 on the pH scale and the capsule should be enteric coated.

GINGIVITIS
See PERIODONTAL DISORDERS.

GLUTEN INTOLERANCE
For many individuals who consume wheat or dairy products, the particular proteins gluten and/or casein are difficult to digest and can lead to intestinal inflammation. When eaten, gluten exhibits a unique amino acid sequence that can create inflammation and a flattening of the villi of the intestinal tract. This becomes a serious disorder since the villi provide the intestine with the ability to absorb nutrients from food. Damaged villi can lead to conditions such as malabsorption, nutrient deficiencies, or even disease, including Celiac disease, leaky gut, or other syndromes.

The main treatment for gluten or casein intolerance has been to remove offending foods from a person's diet, also known as the gluten-free casein-free (GFCF) diet. In the short term, this is effective because a person is removing the proteins that caused the problem, which will reduce inflammation and allow the villi to heal over time. But removing the food does not provide an ultimate solution. If those foods are consumed again, even accidentally, the problems will recur.

Dipeptidyl peptidase is a protein that has multiple functions in the body. When found on the mucosal membrane of the intestinal tract lining, it is known as DPP-IV. DPP-IV is a proteolytic enzyme that is able to break down a particular protein believed to be a contributing factor in gluten and casein intolerance. Though DPP-IV is technically a metabolic enzyme produced by the body, the activity has been discovered in a plant-based protease. Supplements containing plant-based DPP-IV have been used nutritionally with success on individuals with varying levels of sensitivity to gluten and casein.

Formulas that contain DPP-IV along with other proteases offer those suffering from such intolerances an ability to literally digest and assimilate the offending proteins. This proactively heals the gut, reduces inflammation, allows proteins to be properly absorbed in their digested state, and broadens the potential food groups a person may eat. DPP-IV may also be used by those who wish to remain on the GFCF diet to ensure all proteins are broken down safely and effectively.

ENZYME SUPPLEMENTATION SUGGESTIONS:

*High Potency Digestive Formula with every meal

Purpose: To radically enhance the digestion and assimilation of food while reducing the body's need to produce digestive enzymes; the higher potency formula will average about three times the potency of the average digestive formula; an average formula may be substituted if three times the regular dose is taken

Each serving should contain approximately:

Amylase blend	22,000 DU	Alpha-galactosidase	450 GALU
Protease blend	80,000 HUT	Phytase	50 PU
Lipase blend	3,000 FCCFIP	Pectinase	50 AJDU
Cellulase blend	2,000 CU	Xylanase	500 XU
Invertase	80 IAU	Hemicellulase	30 HCU
Lactase	900 LacU	Beta-glucanase	25 BGU
Maltase	200 DP	L. acidophilus	250 million CFU
Glucoamylase	50 AGU		

*DPPIV Formula whenever foods containing gluten are eaten or there is potential that foods eaten have been cooked with foods containing gluten (such as when eating out)

Purpose: To digest gluten (a common allergen found in wheat and cereal grains). DPPIV has proven helpful for individuals who are sensitive to gluten.

Each serving should contain approximately:

DPPIV Protease blend	80,000 HUT	Glucoamylase	15,000 AGU
Amylase blend	15,000 DU		

Soothing Digestive Formula at any time, as needed for discomfort

Purpose: To help alleviate conditions associated with gastrointestinal distress
Each serving should contain approximately:

Amylase blend	2,000 DU	Gotu kola	50 mg
Lipase blend	175 FCCFIP	Papaya leaf	100 mg
Cellulase blend	400 CU	Prickly ash bark	50 mg
Marshmallow root	100 mg		

Additional helpful ingredients:

DGL (deglycyrrhizinated licorice)	

This formula should *not* contain protease. Other herbs may also be present.

GOUT

Gout is a metabolic disorder and a common form of arthritis that is caused by the accumulation of uric acid crystals in the joints. An intensely painful disease, gout most often affects only one joint, typically the big toe, although it can affect other joints, including the ankle, heel, instep, knee, wrist, elbow, or spine. Urate crystals are deposited in tendons, joints, subcutaneous tissue, cartilage, kidneys, and other tissues, and cause inflammation and damage.

Painful gout attacks usually occur at night, may involve fever and chills and are generally preceded by alcohol ingestion, dietary excess, stress, trauma, or certain drugs. Some sources report that gout can be a secondary result of a systemic yeast, fungal infestation, or lead toxicity.

Recommendations include reducing inflammation, eliminating alcohol and high-purine-content foods (meat, fish, lentils, peas, mushrooms, cauliflower) from the diet, reduced consumption of refined carbohydrates and saturated fats, and moderation in protein intake. Other suggestions include increasing intake of cherries and blueberries, which lower uric acid levels; ascertaining the underlying cause of the disorder; and increasing hydration and stress management. Enzymes can be used to reduce inflammation, improve and balance digestion, balance the pH in the body to promote overall health, and support the immune system.

ENZYME SUPPLEMENTATION SUGGESTIONS:

*High Potency Digestive Formula with every meal

Purpose: To radically enhance the digestion and assimilation of food while reducing the body's need to produce digestive enzymes; the higher potency formula will average about three times the potency of the average digestive formula; an average formula may be substituted if three times the regular dose is taken

Each serving should contain approximately:

Amylase blend	22,000 DU	Alpha-galactosidase	450 GALU
Protease blend	80,000 HUT	Phytase	50 PU
Lipase blend	3,000 FCCFIP	Pectinase	50 AJDU
Cellulase blend	2,000 CU	Xylanase	500 XU
Invertase	80 IAU	Hemicellulase	30 HCU
Lactase	900 LacU	Beta-glucanase	25 BGU
Maltase	200 DP	L. acidophilus	250 million CFU
Glucoamylase	50 AGU		

*Anti-inflammatory Formula three times daily or anytime for pain

Purpose: To address inflammation, speed recovery, and repair tissue; best if enteric coated

Each serving should contain approximately:

Protease blend	120,000 HUT	Amylase blend	7,000 DU
Papain	140,000 PU	Lipase blend	600 FCCFIP
Bromelain	1,200 GDU (11.25 million FCCPU)	Catalase	100 baker units

*pH Balancing Formula three times daily between meals

Purpose: To help the body achieve an optimal pH

Each serving should contain approximately:

Amylase blend	25,000 DU	Lipase blend	175 FCCFIP
Cellulase blend	6,000 CU	Pectinase/Phytase	200 PU
Mineral blend	Potassium bicarbonate, sodium bicarbonate, magnesium citrate	Herbal blend	Hydrilla, marshmallow, papaya
Protease blend	1,000 HUT		

The formula should not exceed 8.0 on the pH scale and the capsule should be enteric coated.

High Protease Formula three times daily between meals

Purpose: To help support immune function and assist in removing viruses, fungal forms, toxins, bacteria, and heavy metals
Each capsule should contain approximately:

Protease blend	150,000 HUT	Serratiopeptidase	25,000 units
Mucolase	8 mg	Nattokinase blend	400 FU
Catalase	50 baker units		

Optional: Serratiopeptidase Formula may be added for chronic conditions to relieve pain

Purpose: To break down protein and reduce inflammation. Also supports cardiovascular health and enhances other proteases.
Each serving should contain approximately:

Serratiopeptidase	80,000 SU
Protease blend	70,000 HUT
Mineral blend	50 mg

Supporting enzymes:

Bromelain	Papain

GUM PROBLEMS

See PERIODONTAL DISORDERS.

HAIR LOSS

Loss of hair or baldness may be the expression of your DNA, or it can be caused by many factors, including illness, skin disease, poor diet, poor circulation, diabetes, thyroid disease, surgery, radiation or chemotherapy, pregnancy and the attendant hormonal changes, iron deficiency, drugs, and stress.

Although enzymes may not be able to combat the effects of a genetic predisposition to lose one's hair, they can be used to support the various systems of the body that may be involved with specific causes of hair loss. People who are generally healthy tend to experience less hair loss than people with a variety of health problems. Therefore, using enzymes to support digestion, the absorption of nutrients, the functioning of the immune system, the elimination of free radicals, and balanced pH levels throughout the body can help with this problem.

ENZYME SUPPLEMENTATION SUGGESTIONS:

*High Potency Digestive Formula with every meal

Purpose: To radically enhance the digestion and assimilation of food while reducing the body's need to produce digestive enzymes; the higher potency formula will average about three times the potency of the average digestive formula; an average formula may be substituted if three times the regular dose is taken

Each serving should contain approximately:

Amylase blend	22,000 DU	Alpha-galactosidase	450 GALU
Protease blend	80,000 HUT	Phytase	50 PU
Lipase blend	3,000 FCCFIP	Pectinase	50 AJDU
Cellulase blend	2,000 CU	Xylanase	500 XU
Invertase	80 IAU	Hemicellulase	30 HCU
Lactase	900 LacU	Beta-glucanase	25 BGU
Maltase	200 DP	L. acidophilus	250 million CFU
Glucoamylase	50 AGU		

*High Protease Formula three times daily on an empty stomach

Purpose: To help support immune function and assist in removing viruses, fungal forms, toxins, bacteria, and heavy metals

Each capsule should contain approximately:

Protease blend	150,000 HUT	Serratiopeptidase	25,000 units
Mucolase	8 mg	Nattokinase blend	400 FU
Catalase	50 baker units		

pH Balancing Formula three times daily

Purpose: To help the body achieve an optimal pH

Each serving should contain approximately:

Amylase blend	25,000 DU	Lipase blend	175 FCCFIP
Cellulase blend	6,000 CU	Pectinase/Phytase	200 PU
Mineral blend	Potassium bicarbonate, sodium bicarbonate, magnesium citrate	Herbal blend	Hydrilla, marshmallow, papaya
Protease blend	1,000 HUT		

The formula should not exceed 8.0 on the pH scale and the capsule should be enteric coated.

HALITOSIS

Halitosis is the medical term for bad breath. This condition may be caused by poor digestion, poor oral hygiene, gum disease, tooth decay, constipation, throat or nose infection, liver insufficiencies, inadequate protein digestion, or smoking. It is also often an indication of toxicity of some kind.

A person with persistent halitosis should consult a dentist or a physician to determine if there are any underlying problems that need to be treated. Recommendations for treating halitosis include consistent oral hygiene, healthy diet, and enzyme therapy to improve digestion, support immune function, and balance pH levels. People with this condition may also want to consider the Cleanse and Fortify program described in chapter 4. (See also PERIODONTAL DISORDERS.)

ENZYME SUPPLEMENTATION SUGGESTIONS:

*High Potency Digestive Formula with every meal

Purpose: To radically enhance the digestion and assimilation of food while reducing the body's need to produce digestive enzymes; the higher potency formula will average about three times the potency of the average digestive formula; an average formula may be substituted if three times the regular dose is taken
Each serving should contain approximately:

Amylase blend	22,000 DU	Alpha-galactosidase	450 GALU
Protease blend	80,000 HUT	Phytase	50 PU
Lipase blend	3,000 FCCFIP	Pectinase	50 AJDU
Cellulase blend	2,000 CU	Xylanase	500 XU
Invertase	80 IAU	Hemicellulase	30 HCU
Lactase	900 LacU	Beta-glucanase	25 BGU
Maltase	200 DP	L. acidophilus	250 million CFU
Glucoamylase	50 AGU		

*High Protease Formula three times daily

Purpose: To help support immune function and assist in removing viruses, fungal forms, toxins, bacteria, and heavy metals
Each capsule should contain approximately:

Protease blend	150,000 HUT	Serratiopeptidase	25,000 units
Mucolase	8 mg	Nattokinase blend	400 FU
Catalase	50 baker units		

Probiotic Formula daily before bed

Purpose: To assist the body in balancing microflora

Each serving should contain approximately 5 billion probiotic live cells (guaranteed potency), comprised of:

Bacillus Subtillis	No less than 3 billion CFU guaranteed potency	A blend of *L. acidophilus, L. casei, L. bulgaris, L. plantarum, L. rhamnosus, L. salivarius*	No less than 1 billion CFU guaranteed potency
L. paracassei F-19	No less than 1 billion CFU guaranteed potency		

pH Balancing Formula three times daily

Purpose: To help the body achieve an optimal pH

Each serving should contain approximately:

Amylase blend	25,000 DU	Lipase blend	175 FCCFIP
Cellulase blend	6,000 CU	Pectinase/Phytase	200 PU
Mineral blend	Potassium bicarbonate, sodium bicarbonate, magnesium citrate	Herbal blend	Hydrilla, marshmallow, papaya
Protease blend	1,000 HUT		

The formula should not exceed 8.0 on the pH scale and the capsule should be enteric coated.

Serratiopeptidase Formula three times a day on an empty stomach

Purpose: To break down protein and reduce inflammation. Also supports cardiovascular health and enhances other proteases.

Each serving should contain approximately:

Serratiopeptidase	80,000 SU
Protease blend	70,000 HUT
Mineral blend	50 mg

Supporting enzymes:

Bromelain	Papain

HANGOVER

Hangovers are a result of excessive alcohol consumption, usually beginning sometime after the cessation of consumption, often the next morning. This condition is characterized by headache, nausea, vertigo, diarrhea, and depression. The symptoms are caused by dehydration, imbalanced blood sugar levels, and lowered nutrient levels. The severity of a hangover is determined by the amount and type of alcohol that was consumed.

Besides drinking water, maintaining proper nutrition, and taking supplemental enzymes to treat the symptoms of a hangover, the obvious recommendation is to not overconsume alcohol.

ENZYME SUPPLEMENTATION SUGGESTIONS:

*High Potency Digestive Formula with every meal

Purpose: To radically enhance the digestion and assimilation of food while reducing the body's need to produce digestive enzymes; the higher potency formula will average about three times the potency of the average digestive formula; an average formula may be substituted if three times the regular dose is taken
Each serving should contain approximately:

Amylase blend	22,000 DU	Alpha-galactosidase	450 GALU
Protease blend	80,000 HUT	Phytase	50 PU
Lipase blend	3,000 FCCFIP	Pectinase	50 AJDU
Cellulase blend	2,000 CU	Xylanase	500 XU
Invertase	80 IAU	Hemicellulase	30 HCU
Lactase	900 LacU	Beta-glucanase	25 BGU
Maltase	200 DP	L. acidophilus	250 million CFU
Glucoamylase	50 AGU		

*High Amylase Formula before, during, and after heavy drinking

Purpose: Amylase has been shown to reduce some common symptoms of overconsumption of alcohol, likely because alcohol is converted to sugars in the body.
Each serving should contain approximately:

Amylase blend	22,000 DU	Cellulase blend	400 CU
Glucoamylase	30 AGU	Lactase	300 LacU
Alpha-galactosidase	1,000 GALU	Maltase	300 DP
Protease blend	15,000 HUT	Pectinase	20 endo-PG
Lipase blend	150 FCCFIP		

*High Protease Formula three times daily on empty stomach (more may be taken as needed)

Purpose: To help support immune function and assist in removing viruses, fungal forms, toxins, bacteria, and heavy metals
  Each capsule should contain approximately:

Protease blend	150,000 HUT	Serratiopeptidase	25,000 units
Mucolase	8 mg	Nattokinase blend	400 FU
Catalase	50 baker units		

High Lipase Formula anytime symptoms of dizziness or vertigo occur

Purpose: To reduce symptoms of vertigo
  Each capsule should contain approximately:

Lipase blend	5,000 FCCFIP	Protease blend	20,000 HUT
Amylase blend	10,000 DU	Lactase	300 LacU

Soothing Digestive Formula anytime nauseous

Purpose: To help alleviate conditions associated with gastrointestinal distress
  Each serving should contain approximately:

Amylase blend	2,000 DU	Gotu kola	50 mg
Lipase blend	175 FCCFIP	Papaya leaf	100 mg
Cellulase blend	400 CU	Prickly ash bark	50 mg
Marshmallow root	100 mg		

Additional helpful ingredients:

DGL (deglycyrrhizinated licorice)	

This formula should *not* contain protease. Other herbs may also be present.

HAY FEVER
See ALLERGIES (AIRBORNE).

HEADACHE
Headaches are one of the most common types of pain. The discomfort may be felt throughout the entire head, or may occur in just one area. It may last for thirty

minutes or for days. The attributes of a headache typically depend upon the type or cause of the pain. Many headaches are the body's response to an adverse stimulus, such as hunger, stress, dehydration, or an allergen. But headaches can also be caused by illness, pollution, caffeine, alcohol, sulfites, fatigue, fever, drugs, constipation, toxins, vitamin deficiencies, poor vertebral alignment, hypertension, meningitis, head injury, tumor, vision or eye problems, or serious injury or illness. Many headaches are caused by unknown or undetermined factors.

There are four common types of headaches. Tension headaches are caused by a tightening in the muscles of the face, neck, shoulders, and scalp or muscle spasms in these areas, usually due to fatigue or stress. A migraine is a severe, incapacitating headache usually preceded or accompanied by visual disturbances, light sensitivity, and nausea or vomiting. Migraines are caused by constriction of the arteries that lead to the brain, although there are a variety of possible underlying causes. (See MIGRAINES.) Cluster headaches, a type of migraine, typically cause severe pain around or behind one eye. Sinus headaches are caused by congestion and possibly infection of the sinuses. The pain is usually in the face, spreading from above the eyes to as far as the gum line. A feeling of pressure is common.

Persistent headaches without a specific cause may be due to your environment or food intake. In this case, start with the Cleanse and Fortify Program described in chapter 4 to bring your body back into balance. After a few days, continue with the Optimal Nutrient Support program to ensure good health.

Recommendations for treating headaches include determining the underlying cause of the headaches and avoiding exposure to any known trigger; stress management; getting enough rest; and using enzymes to support the digestive and immune systems and reduce inflammation that may be associated with the headache.

IMPORTANT NOTE: *In the event that your headache is accompanied by blurred vision, heart pounding, visual color changes, sensitivity to light, pressure behind the eyes that is relieved by vomiting, or was the result of a blow or an injury to the head, consult with your physician immediately.*

ENZYME SUPPLEMENTATION SUGGESTIONS:

*High Potency Digestive Formula with every meal

Purpose: To radically enhance the digestion and assimilation of food while reducing the body's need to produce digestive enzymes; the higher potency formula will average about three times the potency of the average digestive formula; an average formula may be substituted if three times the regular dose is taken

Each serving should contain approximately:

Amylase blend	22,000 DU	Alpha-galactosidase	450 GALU
Protease blend	80,000 HUT	Phytase	50 PU
Lipase blend	3,000 FCCFIP	Pectinase	50 AJDU
Cellulase blend	2,000 CU	Xylanase	500 XU
Invertase	80 IAU	Hemicellulase	30 HCU
Lactase	900 LacU	Beta-glucanase	25 BGU
Maltase	200 DP	*L. acidophilus*	250 million CFU
Glucoamylase	50 AGU		

*Anti-inflammatory Formula three times daily or anytime needed for pain

Purpose: To address inflammation, speed recovery, and repair tissue; best if enteric coated

Each serving should contain approximately:

Protease blend	120,000 HUT	Amylase blend	7,000 DU
Papain	140,000 PU	Lipase blend	600 FCCFIP
Bromelain	1,200 GDU (11.25 million FCCPU)	Catalase	100 baker units

*Serratiopeptidase Formula three times daily or anytime needed for pain

Purpose: To break down protein and reduce inflammation. Also supports cardiovascular health and enhances other proteases.

Each serving should contain approximately:

Serratiopeptidase	80,000 SU
Protease blend	70,000 HUT
Mineral blend	50 mg

Supporting enzymes:

Bromelain	Papain

HEARTBURN

See GASTROESOPHAGEAL REFLUX DISEASE.

HEMORRHOIDS

Hemorrhoids are varicose (swollen or inflamed) veins in the rectum (internal hemorrhoids) and anus (external hemorrhoids). Hemorrhoids can bleed when irritated and can cause pain and itching. Hemorrhoids are typically caused by pressure on the veins in the rectum and anus. Factors that can cause the development of hemorrhoids include constipation, poor diet, lack of adequate fluids, lack of exercise, pregnancy, allergies, liver damage, long periods of sitting on hard surfaces, and tumors or cysts in the colon or rectum. Severe hemorrhoids may require surgery.

Recommendations include determining the cause of the condition, increasing fiber and fluids in the diet, establishing bowel regularity, and supplementation with enzymes to treat constipation and aid in the healing process by improving circulation.

ENZYME SUPPLEMENTATION SUGGESTIONS:

*High Potency Digestive Formula with every meal

Purpose: To radically enhance the digestion and assimilation of food while reducing the body's need to produce digestive enzymes; the higher potency formula will average about three times the potency of the average digestive formula; an average formula may be substituted if three times the regular dose is taken
Each serving should contain approximately:

Amylase blend	22,000 DU	Alpha-galactosidase	450 GALU
Protease blend	80,000 HUT	Phytase	50 PU
Lipase blend	3,000 FCCFIP	Pectinase	50 AJDU
Cellulase blend	2,000 CU	Xylanase	500 XU
Invertase	80 IAU	Hemicellulase	30 HCU
Lactase	900 LacU	Beta-glucanase	25 BGU
Maltase	200 DP	L. acidophilus	250 million CFU
Glucoamylase	50 AGU		

*Nattokinase Formula three times daily

Purpose: To decrease blood pressure and increase circulation by breaking down fibrin

Each serving should contain approximately:
Necessary ingredient:

Nattokinase NSK-SD	1,000 FU

Helpful ingredients:

Amylase blend	9,000 DU	Glucoamylase	25 AGU
Protease blend	20,000 HUT	Lipase blend	1,000 FCCFIP
Minerals	85 mg	Cellulase blend	400 CU

High Cellulase Formula three times daily between meals for one week

Purpose: To manage yeast overgrowth
Each capsule should contain approximately:

Cellulase blend	30,000 CU
Protease blend	100,000 HUT

Contraindications: High amounts of cellulase should not be taken with certain timed-release medications that contain cellulose.

HERPES VIRUS

The herpes virus is a recurrent viral infection of the skin and mucous membranes. It is characterized by small, often painful watery blisters that occur around the mouth, lips, genitals, conjunctivae, and corneas. Eventually the blisters may break, crust over, and form small ulcers in the skin or affected area.

There are two types of herpes virus. Herpes type I involves skin eruptions, cold sores, or fever blisters. It can also cause inflammation of the cornea, which, if left untreated, can cause encephalitis. Herpes type II (also called genital herpes) is the most prevalent herpes infection. Sexually transmitted, it affects the genitals, involving painful blisters that develop on and around the genitalia in both men and women. The blisters, which later develop into painful ulcers, are often accompanied by painful urination, swelling, and a urethral discharge. Both men and women may experience swollen lymph nodes in the region, muscular aches, and a low-grade fever during outbreaks.

The herpes virus becomes dormant in the nerve cells in most individuals after the initial infection. Other individuals, however, can experience recurrent outbreaks. Type I has a recurrence rate of 4 percent, while Type II has a 60 percent recurrence rate. Recurrent outbreaks may follow stress, sun exposure, minor infections, and trauma. The incubation period for this contagious virus is two to twelve days.

Recommendations include reducing dietary toxicity, reducing emotional and environmental stress, and using enzyme therapy to provide optimum support to the immune system, improve digestion and nutrient uptake, and balance pH levels.

ENZYME SUPPLEMENTATION SUGGESTIONS:

*High Potency Digestive Formula with every meal

Purpose: To radically enhance the digestion and assimilation of food while reducing the body's need to produce digestive enzymes; the higher potency formula will average about three times the potency of the average digestive formula; an average formula may be substituted if three times the regular dose is taken
Each serving should contain approximately:

Amylase blend	22,000 DU	Alpha-galactosidase	450 GALU
Protease blend	80,000 HUT	Phytase	50 PU
Lipase blend	3,000 FCCFIP	Pectinase	50 AJDU
Cellulase blend	2,000 CU	Xylanase	500 XU
Invertase	80 IAU	Hemicellulase	30 HCU
Lactase	900 LacU	Beta-glucanase	25 BGU
Maltase	200 DP	L. acidophilus	250 million CFU
Glucoamylase	50 AGU		

*High Protease Formula three times daily between meals

Purpose: To help support immune function and assist in removing viruses, fungal forms, toxins, bacteria, and heavy metals
Each capsule should contain approximately:

Protease blend	150,000 HUT	Serratiopeptidase	25,000 units
Mucolase	8 mg	Nattokinase blend	400 FU
Catalase	50 baker units		

pH Balancing Formula two times daily, morning and night

Purpose: To help the body achieve an optimal pH
Each serving should contain approximately:

Amylase blend	25,000 DU	Lipase blend	175 FCCFIP
Cellulase blend	6,000 CU	Pectinase/Phytase	200 PU
Mineral blend	Potassium bicarbonate, sodium bicarbonate, magnesium citrate	Herbal blend	Hydrilla, marshmallow, papaya
Protease blend	1,000 HUT		

The formula should not exceed 8.0 on the pH scale and the capsule should be enteric coated.

HERPES ZOSTER (SHINGLES)

Herpes zoster, or shingles, is a relatively common infection of the nerves of the skin. The most serious feature of the virus is the pain that follows a rash of small, crusting blisters. After the rash heals, the pain may persist for months, or even years, as a consequence of damage to the nerves. It is possible to reduce the severity of the active stage and to minimize nerve damage by the prompt use of antiviral drugs.

Herpes zoster is actually caused by the varicella-zoster virus, which also causes chicken pox. After someone recovers from chicken pox, most of the viral organisms are destroyed, but some survive and lay dormant in certain sensory nerves. A decline in the efficiency of the immune system allows the viruses to reemerge and cause shingles.

Herpes zoster can occur due to stress or because the immune system has been weakened, either by disease, such as lymphoma or Hodgkin's disease, or by treatment with immunosuppressant or anticancer drugs. The first indication of a herpes zoster outbreak is excessive sensitivity in the affected area of skin, soon followed by pain, and then (after about five days) a rash, which may leave scars after crusting.

People who have herpes zoster should see a doctor immediately. Additional recommendations include reducing dietary toxicity, reducing emotional and environmental stress, and using enzymes to provide optimum support of the immune and digestive systems, balance pH levels, and reduce inflammation and pain during the outbreak of the rash.

ENZYME SUPPLEMENTATION SUGGESTIONS:

*High Potency Digestive Formula with every meal

Purpose: To radically enhance the digestion and assimilation of food while reducing the body's need to produce digestive enzymes; the higher potency formula will average about three times the potency of the average digestive formula; an average formula may be substituted if three times the regular dose is taken

Each serving should contain approximately:

Amylase blend	22,000 DU	Alpha-galactosidase	450 GALU
Protease blend	80,000 HUT	Phytase	50 PU
Lipase blend	3,000 FCCFIP	Pectinase	50 AJDU
Cellulase blend	2,000 CU	Xylanase	500 XU
Invertase	80 IAU	Hemicellulase	30 HCU
Lactase	900 LacU	Beta-glucanase	25 BGU
Maltase	200 DP	L. acidophilus	250 million CFU
Glucoamylase	50 AGU		

*High Protease Formula three times per day, increase to four times per day at outbreak

Purpose: To help support immune function and assist in removing viruses, fungal forms, toxins, bacteria, and heavy metals
   Each capsule should contain approximately:

Protease blend	150,000 HUT	Serratiopeptidase	25,000 units
Mucolase	8 mg	Nattokinase blend	400 FU
Catalase	50 baker units		

Serratiopeptidase Formula three times a day on an empty stomach

Purpose: To break down protein and reduce inflammation. Also supports cardiovascular health and enhances other proteases.
   Each serving should contain approximately:

Serratiopeptidase	80,000 SU
Protease blend	70,000 HUT
Mineral blend	50 mg

Supporting enzymes:

Bromelain	Papain

pH Balancing Formula three times daily

Purpose: To help the body achieve an optimal pH
Each serving should contain approximately:

Amylase blend	25,000 DU	Lipase blend	175 FCCFIP
Cellulase blend	6,000 CU	Pectinase/Phytase	200 PU
Mineral blend	Potassium bicarbonate, sodium bicarbonate, magnesium citrate	Herbal blend	Hydrilla, marshmallow, papaya
Protease blend	1,000 HUT		

The formula should not exceed 8.0 on the pH scale and the capsule should be enteric coated.

Optional: Anti-inflammatory Formula may be added during outbreak

Purpose: To address inflammation, speed recovery, and repair tissue; best if enteric coated
Each serving should contain approximately:

Protease blend	120,000 HUT	Amylase blend	7,000 DU
Papain	140,000 PU	Lipase blend	600 FCCFIP
Bromelain	1,200 GDU (11.25 million FCCPU)	Catalase	100 baker units

HIATAL HERNIA

A hiatal hernia is the protrusion (or hernia) of the upper part of the stomach into the thorax through a tear, opening, or weakness (hiatus) in the diaphragm. The muscle at the end of the esophagus may be affected, which can cause acid reflux (regurgitation of acidic gastric juices into the esophagus). (See GASTROESOPHA-GEAL REFLUX.) This reflux, in turn, may cause heartburn and belching that may be made worse by either bending or lying down. Very large hiatal hernias sometimes require surgical repair.

Recommendations include avoiding large, heavy meals; supplementing the diet with digestive enzymes to promote efficient and complete digestion and absorption of foods; and raising the head off the bed to keep the upper body in a raised position during sleep.

ENZYME SUPPLEMENTATION SUGGESTIONS:

*High Potency Digestive Formula with every meal

Purpose: To radically enhance the digestion and assimilation of food while reducing the body's need to produce digestive enzymes; the higher potency formula will average about three times the potency of the average digestive formula; an average formula may be substituted if three times the regular dose is taken
Each serving should contain approximately:

Amylase blend	22,000 DU	Alpha-galactosidase	450 GALU
Protease blend	80,000 HUT	Phytase	50 PU
Lipase blend	3,000 FCCFIP	Pectinase	50 AJDU
Cellulase blend	2,000 CU	Xylanase	500 XU
Invertase	80 IAU	Hemicellulase	30 HCU
Lactase	900 LacU	Beta-glucanase	25 BGU
Maltase	200 DP	*L. acidophilus*	250 million CFU
Glucoamylase	50 AGU		

*Soothing Digestive Formula after every meal and as needed for discomfort

Purpose: To help alleviate conditions associated with gastrointestinal distress
Each serving should contain approximately:

Amylase blend	2,000 DU	Gotu kola	50 mg
Lipase blend	175 FCCFIP	Papaya leaf	100 mg
Cellulase blend	400 CU	Prickly ash bark	50 mg
Marshmallow root	100 mg		

Additional helpful ingredients:

DGL (deglycyrrhizinated licorice)	

This formula should *not* contain protease. Other herbs may also be present.

HIGH BLOOD PRESSURE
See HYPERTENSION.

HOT FLASHES
See MENOPAUSE.

HORMONAL IMBALANCES
See ENDOCRINE GLANDS.

HYPERTENSION

Hypertension is the clinical term for high blood pressure. Blood pressure is the pressure exerted by the blood against the walls of the blood vessels. There are two measures of blood pressure. Systolic pressure measures the pressure when the heart contracts and forces blood into the arteries. This is the higher number in a typical blood pressure reading. Diastolic pressure is the pressure in the blood vessels when the heart relaxes. This is typically the lower number. A diastolic measure over 90 and a systolic measure over 140 is usually considered high.

Hypertension can be caused by a variety of factors, including stress, kidney disease, high cholesterol that congests the arteries, and hardening of the arteries. Factors that increase the risk of this disorder include smoking, obesity, excessive use of stimulants and caffeine, drug abuse, use of birth control pills, and a high sodium/low potassium intake.

Mild hypertension may respond to weight or stress reduction, but more severe forms may require additional lifestyle changes and possibly treatment with prescription medications. For most people, treatment should include exercise. Regular activity has a number of proven, positive health effects, especially on heart health. Vigorous exercise strengthens the heart as a pump, making it a larger, more efficient muscle. Even moderate activity can boost HDL "good" cholesterol, aid the circulatory system, and lower blood pressure and blood fats. All these effects translate into reduced risk for heart disease, heart attack, and stroke.

Other recommendations include diagnostic tests and evaluations to determine the underlying cause of the hypertension, supplementing the diet with minerals to correct mineral deficiencies, and enzyme therapy to improve digestion and nutrient absorption and to improve circulation, lower blood pressure, and improve cardiovascular health.

ENZYME SUPPLEMENTATION SUGGESTIONS:

*High Potency Digestive Formula with every meal

Purpose: To radically enhance the digestion and assimilation of food while reducing the body's need to produce digestive enzymes; the higher potency formula will average about three times the potency of the average digestive formula; an average formula may be substituted if three times the regular dose is taken

Each serving should contain approximately:

Amylase blend	22,000 DU	Alpha-galactosidase	450 GALU
Protease blend	80,000 HUT	Phytase	50 PU
Lipase blend	3,000 FCCFIP	Pectinase	50 AJDU
Cellulase blend	2,000 CU	Xylanase	500 XU
Invertase	80 IAU	Hemicellulase	30 HCU
Lactase	900 LacU	Beta-glucanase	25 BGU
Maltase	200 DP	L. acidophilus	250 million CFU
Glucoamylase	50 AGU		

*Nattokinase Formula three times daily between meals

Purpose: To support cardiovascular health and decrease blood pressure by breaking down fibrin

Each serving should contain approximately:
Necessary ingredient:

Nattokinase NSK-SD	1,000 FU

Helpful ingredients:

Amylase blend	9,000 DU	Glucoamylase	25 AGU
Protease blend	20,000 HUT	Lipase blend	1,000 FCCFIP
Minerals	85 mg	Cellulase blend	400 CU

*High Lipase Formula three times a day on an empty stomach

Purpose: To improve fat digestion and metabolism, as well as the health of the cardiovascular system

Each capsule should contain approximately:

Lipase blend	5,000 FCCFIP	Protease blend	20,000 HUT
Amylase blend	10,000 DU	Lactase	300 LacU

HYPOGLYCEMIA

Hypoglycemia is a condition characterized by low glucose (blood sugar) levels. When blood sugar levels are low, various systems in the body are affected. The principle symptoms arise from an inadequate supply of glucose as fuel for the brain, resulting in an impairment of function. This condition refers to a blood glucose level below 70 milligrams per deciliter for the typical patient, although the number doctors consider "low" varies depending upon the characteristics of the patient. Some experts suggest that it is not a low blood sugar count per se that causes the symptoms of hypoglycemia, but rather the rapid fall of blood sugar levels.

There are two categories of hypoglycemia: drug-related and nondrug-related. Drug-related hypoglycemia is the most common and occurs in people taking medication or insulin in the treatment of diabetes. Nondrug-related hypoglycemia is less common. There are two types of nondrug-related hypoglycemia: fasting and reactive. Fasting hypoglycemia is usually related to an underlying disease or disorder. Reactive hypoglycemia is marked by symptoms that develop three to five hours after meals and are relieved by eating, and is not related to any underlying disorder.

Symptoms of hypoglycemia can include one or more of the following: anxiety, irritability, headache, depression, trembling, excessive sweating, palpitations, confusion, double vision, weakness, bizarre behavior, incoherent speech, and convulsions.

The primary goal in hypoglycemia management is to reestablish healthy blood sugar control. One method is through dietary therapy encouraging frequent small meals. In addition, all processed, concentrated simple carbohydrates and alcohol should be avoided. Regular exercise is also important. Enzymes can improve the digestive process, particularly the digestion of sugars, and raise glucose levels between meals.

ENZYME SUPPLEMENTATION SUGGESTIONS:

High Potency Digestive Formula or **High Amylase Formula** with every meal

Purpose: To radically enhance the digestion and assimilation of food while reducing the body's need to produce digestive enzymes; the higher potency formula will average about three times the potency of the average digestive formula; an average formula may be substituted if three times the regular dose is taken

Each serving should contain approximately:

Amylase blend	22,000 DU	Alpha-galactosidase	450 GALU
Protease blend	80,000 HUT	Phytase	50 PU
Lipase blend	3,000 FCCFIP	Pectinase	50 AJDU
Cellulase blend	2,000 CU	Xylanase	500 XU
Invertase	80 IAU	Hemicellulase	30 HCU
Lactase	900 LacU	Beta-glucanase	25 BGU
Maltase	200 DP	*L. acidophilus*	250 million CFU
Glucoamylase	50 AGU		

High Amylase Formula three times daily or as needed between meals to raise glucose levels and break down excess sugars

Purpose: To overcome symptoms of allergies and for the proper digestion of carbohydrates, especially grains, raw vegetables, and legumes

Each serving should contain approximately:

Amylase blend	22,000 DU	Cellulase blend	400 CU
Glucoamylase	30 AGU	Lactase	300 LacU
Alpha-galactosidase	1,000 GALU	Maltase	300 DP
Protease blend	15,000 HUT	Pectinase	20 endo-PG
Lipase blend	150 FCCFIP		

HYPOTHYROIDISM

Hypothyroidism is a disease state caused by insufficient production of thyroid hormone by the thyroid gland. An insufficiency in thyroid hormones can have an effect on all body functions, but particularly affects the metabolic rate. A deficiency generally results in a large array of signs and symptoms. These can include fatigue; weight gain; weakness; depression; infertility; constipation; low basal body temperature (below 97.6); thin, brittle nails; hair loss; rough, dry skin; muscle weakness; forgetfulness; difficulty concentrating; joint stiffness; prolonged and heavy menstrual bleeding; cold hands and feet; sluggish lymphatic drainage; impaired kidney function; and increased risks of heart disease, hypertension, and atherosclerosis.

Hypothyroidism can be caused by thyroid surgery (removal of part of the gland due to tumors or cysts), an autoimmune disease that causes the body to attack the gland (Hashimoto's disease), radiation therapy to treat cancer or hyperthyroidism, medications, a pituitary disorder, or an iodine deficiency. Most cases of hypothyroidism are not present at birth, but develop in adults. Advanced hypothyroidism may cause severe complications.

Recommendations for hypothyroidism include maintaining a well-balanced diet, getting regular exercise, and possibly using a synthetic thyroid supplement or a natural supplement derived from animal thyroid to stimulate thyroid gland secretion. Enzymes can be used to improve digestion, particularly the digestion of fats and carbohydrates; improve energy levels; and support proper functioning of the endocrine system and organs.

ENZYME SUPPLEMENTATION SUGGESTIONS:

*High Potency Digestive Formula with every meal

Purpose: To radically enhance the digestion and assimilation of food while reducing the body's need to produce digestive enzymes; the higher potency formula will average about three times the potency of the average digestive formula; an average formula may be substituted if three times the regular dose is taken

Each serving should contain approximately:

Amylase blend	22,000 DU	Alpha-galactosidase	450 GALU
Protease blend	80,000 HUT	Phytase	50 PU
Lipase blend	3,000 FCCFIP	Pectinase	50 AJDU
Cellulase blend	2,000 CU	Xylanase	500 XU
Invertase	80 IAU	Hemicellulase	30 HCU
Lactase	900 LacU	Beta-glucanase	25 BGU
Maltase	200 DP	L. acidophilus	250 million CFU
Glucoamylase	50 AGU		

*High Lipase Formula three times daily between meals

Purpose: To improve fat digestion and metabolism, as well as the health of the cardiovascular system

Each capsule should contain approximately:

Lipase blend	5,000 FCCFIP	Protease blend	20,000 HUT
Amylase blend	10,000 DU	Lactase	300 LacU

High Amylase Formula may be added to help increase energy level

Purpose: To overcome symptoms of allergies and for the proper digestion of carbohydrates, especially grains, raw vegetables, and legumes

Each serving should contain approximately:

Amylase blend	22,000 DU	Cellulase blend	400 CU
Glucoamylase	30 AGU	Lactase	300 LacU
Alpha-galactosidase	1,000 GALU	Maltase	300 DP
Protease blend	15,000 HUT	Pectinase	20 endo-PG
Lipase blend	150 FCCFIP		

High Protease Formula three times per day for detoxification and organ support

Purpose: To help support immune function and assist in removing viruses, fungal forms, toxins, bacteria, and heavy metals

Each capsule should contain approximately:

Protease blend	150,000 HUT	Serratiopeptidase	25,000 units
Mucolase	8 mg	Nattokinase blend	400 FU
Catalase	50 baker units		

INDIGESTION

Indigestion is a condition that is frequently caused by eating too fast (especially high-fat or spicy foods), eating without chewing properly, overeating, and eating while under stress or when tired. Food that has been badly cooked or overprocessed can also promote indigestion. Food allergies, enzyme deficiencies, irritation of the stomach, too much or too little stomach acid, and changes in diet (even for the better) can all cause indigestion.

Symptoms may include heartburn (see also GASTROESOPHAGEAL REFLUX), bloating, nausea, FLATULENCE, belching, cramps, a disagreeable taste in the mouth, and sometimes vomiting and diarrhea. Over time, indigestion can lead to more serious problems, including stress on the immune system, lack of proper digestive enzymes, and poor nutrient absorption.

Recommendations include eating a well-balanced, healthy diet; thoroughly chewing food; eating in a comfortable, relaxed environment; and avoiding drinking large quantities of water during meals. Enzymes can be used to improve digestion and nutrient absorption, soothe the digestive tract, support the immune system, and balance the pH levels in the body.

ENZYME SUPPLEMENTATION SUGGESTIONS:

*High Potency Digestive Formula with every meal

Purpose: To radically enhance the digestion and assimilation of food while reducing the body's need to produce digestive enzymes; the higher potency formula will average about three times the potency of the average digestive formula; an average formula may be substituted if three times the regular dose is taken

Each serving should contain approximately:

Amylase blend	22,000 DU	Alpha-galactosidase	450 GALU
Protease blend	80,000 HUT	Phytase	50 PU
Lipase blend	3,000 FCCFIP	Pectinase	50 AJDU
Cellulase blend	2,000 CU	Xylanase	500 XU
Invertase	80 IAU	Hemicellulase	30 HCU
Lactase	900 LacU	Beta-glucanase	25 BGU
Maltase	200 DP	L. acidophilus	250 million CFU
Glucoamylase	50 AGU		

*Soothing Digestive Formula after meals

Purpose: To help alleviate conditions associated with gastrointestinal distress
Each serving should contain approximately:

Amylase blend	2,000 DU	Gotu kola	50 mg
Lipase blend	175 FCCFIP	Papaya leaf	100 mg
Cellulase blend	400 CU	Prickly ash bark	50 mg
Marshmallow root	100 mg		

Additional helpful ingredients:

DGL (deglycyrrhizinated licorice)	

This formula should *not* contain protease. Other herbs may also be present.

Optional: pH Balancing Formula two times daily

Purpose: To help the body achieve an optimal pH
Each serving should contain approximately:

Amylase blend	25,000 DU	Lipase blend	175 FCCFIP
Cellulase blend	6,000 CU	Pectinase/Phytase	200 PU
Mineral blend	Potassium bicarbonate, sodium bicarbonate, magnesium citrate	Herbal blend	Hydrilla, marshmallow, papaya
Protease blend	1,000 HUT		

The formula should not exceed 8.0 on the pH scale and the capsule should be enteric coated.

INFECTION

Disease-causing microorganisms (such as bacteria, viruses, and fungi) can establish opportunistic colonies in and on the human body. An infection is the detrimental colonization of a host organism by a foreign species, multiplying at the expense of the host. The host's first response to infection is inflammation, as the body attempts to control and eliminate these microorganisms. This process increases the flow of blood to the infected area, bringing white blood cells and other components of the immune system to attack the invading microorganisms.

Symptoms of infection can include an elevated temperature, redness, pain, swelling, and the formation of pus. Infections must be treated by a medical professional, but enzymes can be used to help the body fight the infection by supporting the digestive system and increasing nutrient absorption, strengthening the immune system, reducing inflammation and pain, and balancing pH levels.

ENZYME SUPPLEMENTATION SUGGESTIONS:

*High Potency Digestive Formula with every meal

Purpose: To radically enhance the digestion and assimilation of food while reducing the body's need to produce digestive enzymes; the higher potency formula will average about three times the potency of the average digestive formula; an average formula may be substituted if three times the regular dose is taken
Each serving should contain approximately:

Amylase blend	22,000 DU	Alpha-galactosidase	450 GALU
Protease blend	80,000 HUT	Phytase	50 PU
Lipase blend	3,000 FCCFIP	Pectinase	50 AJDU
Cellulase blend	2,000 CU	Xylanase	500 XU
Invertase	80 IAU	Hemicellulase	30 HCU
Lactase	900 LacU	Beta-glucanase	25 BGU
Maltase	200 DP	L. acidophilus	250 million CFU
Glucoamylase	50 AGU		

*High Protease Formula three times daily

Purpose: To help support immune function and assist in removing viruses, fungal forms, toxins, bacteria, and heavy metals
Each capsule should contain approximately:

Protease blend	150,000 HUT	Serratiopeptidase	25,000 units
Mucolase	8 mg	Nattokinase blend	400 FU
Catalase	50 baker units		

Anti-inflammatory Formula anytime for pain or inflammation

Purpose: To address inflammation, speed recovery, and repair tissue; best if enteric coated

Each serving should contain approximately:

Protease blend	120,000 HUT	Amylase blend	7,000 DU
Papain	140,000 PU	Lipase blend	600 FCCFIP
Bromelain	1,200 GDU (11.25 million FCCPU)	Catalase	100 baker units

Optional: pH Balancing Formula three times daily

Purpose: To help the body achieve an optimal pH

Each serving should contain approximately:

Amylase blend	25,000 DU	Lipase blend	175 FCCFIP
Cellulase blend	6,000 CU	Pectinase/Phytase	200 PU
Mineral blend	Potassium bicarbonate, sodium bicarbonate, magnesium citrate	Herbal blend	Hydrilla, marshmallow, papaya
Protease blend	1,000 HUT		

The formula should not exceed 8.0 on the pH scale and the capsule should be enteric coated.

INFLAMMATORY BOWEL DISEASE

There are two common types of inflammatory bowel disease. Ulcerative colitis is an inflammation of the mucous membranes of the colon (large intestine) and rectum. Poor eating habits (diets high in fat and processed foods), food allergies, viral or bacterial infection, and genetic makeup may be possible causes of colitis, though there are no clear, defined causes. The symptoms include severe abdominal cramps and diarrhea (usually with blood and mucus) and sometimes fever.

Crohn's Disease, a less common ailment, is a chronic inflammatory disease that can affect any part of the gastrointestinal tract, from the mouth to the anus. The intestinal wall becomes extremely thick due to chronic inflammation. As the inflamed areas heal, scar tissue can narrow the intestinal passageway. This condition may cause pain, fever, diarrhea (sometimes bloody), weight loss, abdominal pain, malabsorption, anemia, and fatigue. The cause of Crohn's Disease is still unknown; however, the risk increases with a history of food allergies.

A diet rich in fresh vegetables, fruit, and good sources of protein is suggested to reduce the risk of a breakout, minimize ill effects, and reduce the chances of contracting these diseases. Too many starches, fats, red meat, or dairy products may irritate the colon. Regular physical activity is very important to keep the gastrointestinal tract functioning normally. Recommendations also include an elimination diet to rule out food allergens, increased hydration, relaxation to reduce stress, and supplemental digestive enzymes, probiotics, and nutrients to support healthy digestion, strengthen the immune system, and promote balanced pH levels. Enzymes can also be used to reduce the inflammation in the colon.

ENZYME SUPPLEMENTATION SUGGESTIONS:

*High Potency Digestive Formula with meals

Purpose: To radically enhance the digestion and assimilation of food while reducing the body's need to produce digestive enzymes; the higher potency formula will average about three times the potency of the average digestive formula; an average formula may be substituted if three times the regular dose is taken
Each serving should contain approximately:

Amylase blend	22,000 DU	Alpha-galactosidase	450 GALU
Protease blend	80,000 HUT	Phytase	50 PU
Lipase blend	3,000 FCCFIP	Pectinase	50 AJDU
Cellulase blend	2,000 CU	Xylanase	500 XU
Invertase	80 IAU	Hemicellulase	30 HCU
Lactase	900 LacU	Beta-glucanase	25 BGU
Maltase	200 DP	L. acidophilus	250 million CFU
Glucoamylase	50 AGU		

*Soothing Digestive Formula after each meal

Purpose: To help alleviate conditions associated with gastrointestinal distress
Each serving should contain approximately:

Amylase blend	2,000 DU	Gotu kola	50 mg
Lipase blend	175 FCCFIP	Papaya leaf	100 mg
Cellulase blend	400 CU	Prickly ash bark	50 mg
Marshmallow root	100 mg		

Additional helpful ingredients:

DGL (deglycyrrhizinated licorice)	

This formula should *not* contain protease. Other herbs may also be present.

*Probiotic Formula daily before bed

Purpose: To assist the body in balancing microflora
　　Each serving should contain approximately 5 billion probiotic live cells (guaranteed potency), comprised of:

Bacillus Subtillis	No less than 3 billion CFU guaranteed potency	A blend of *L. acidophilus, L. casei, L. bulgaris, L. plantarum, L. rhamnosus, L. salivarius*	No less than 1 billion CFU guaranteed potency
L. paracassei F-19	No less than 1 billion CFU guaranteed potency		

Anti-inflammatory Formula three times daily (or anytime inflammation occurs)

Purpose: To address inflammation, speed recovery, and repair tissue; best if enteric coated
　　Each serving should contain approximately:

Protease blend	120,000 HUT	Amylase blend	7,000 DU
Papain	140,000 PU	Lipase blend	600 FCCFIP
Bromelain	1,200 GDU (11.25 million FCCPU)	Catalase	100 baker units

pH Balancing Formula three times daily

Purpose: To help the body achieve an optimal pH
　　Each serving should contain approximately:

Amylase blend	25,000 DU	Lipase blend	175 FCCFIP
Cellulase blend	6,000 CU	Pectinase/Phytase	200 PU
Mineral blend	Potassium bicarbonate, sodium bicarbonate, magnesium citrate	Herbal blend	Hydrilla, marshmallow, papaya
Protease blend	1,000 HUT		

　　The formula should not exceed 8.0 on the pH scale and the capsule should be enteric coated.

INFLUENZA

Influenza, commonly called the flu, is a highly contagious viral infection of the respiratory tract (the lungs and airways). The symptoms of flu include fever, chills, runny nose, sore throat, cough, headache, gastrointestinal disturbances, lack of appetite, muscle aches, nerve pain, extreme fatigue, and a general feeling of malaise. Coughing and sneezing can spread this common ailment. The incubation period is one to three days. Influenza may also increase susceptibility to pneumonia, sinus problems, ear infections, and other bacterial and viral infections because it weakens the immune system.

Recommendations include seeking treatment from a medical professional if you are at risk for further complications (if you are elderly, are immunosuppressed, or have cardiovascular or pulmonary disease). If you are not at risk, recommendations include increasing hydration, rest, support of the immune and digestive systems, and reducing mucus production.

ENZYME SUPPLEMENTATION SUGGESTIONS:
*High Protease Formula three to four times per day

Purpose: To help support immune function and assist in removing viruses, fungal forms, toxins, bacteria, and heavy metals
Each capsule should contain approximately:

Protease blend	150,000 HUT	Serratiopeptidase	25,000 units
Mucolase	8 mg	Nattokinase blend	400 FU
Catalase	50 baker units		

*Mucolase Formula three times daily for symptom relief

Purpose: To reduce excess mucus produced by the body; particularly helpful in treating sinus and chest congestion
Each serving should contain approximately:

Mucolase	30 mg

Supporting enzymes:

Amylase blend	7,000 DU	Cellulase blend	200 CU
Protease blend	20,000 HUT	Xylanase	250 XU
Glucoamylase	25 AGU	Pectinase with Phytase	175 endo-PG
Beta-glucanase	30 BGU	Hemicellulase	30 HCU
Lipase blend	250 FCCFIP	Invertase	5 INVU
Alpha-galactosidase	50 GALU		

High Potency Digestive Formula with every meal

Purpose: To radically enhance the digestion and assimilation of food while reducing the body's need to produce digestive enzymes; the higher potency formula will average about three times the potency of the average digestive formula; an average formula may be substituted if three times the regular dose is taken

Each serving should contain approximately:

Amylase blend	22,000 DU	Alpha-galactosidase	450 GALU
Protease blend	80,000 HUT	Phytase	50 PU
Lipase blend	3,000 FCCFIP	Pectinase	50 AJDU
Cellulase blend	2,000 CU	Xylanase	500 XU
Invertase	80 IAU	Hemicellulase	30 HCU
Lactase	900 LacU	Beta-glucanase	25 BGU
Maltase	200 DP	L. acidophilus	250 million CFU
Glucoamylase	50 AGU		

INSECT BITES AND STINGS

All insect bites provoke a reaction in the skin that is primarily an allergic response to substances in the insect's saliva, venom, or deposited feces. A honeybee's stinger is barbed and remains in the wound. The bee sting sac is rich in sugars. The wasp sting is primarily the stomach organ and the stinger of the wasp, which is comprised of protein. Many spider venoms are composed of complex proteins and proteolytic enzymes.

Enzymes can be used as a salve and systemically to combat the effects of bites and stings. When using the enzymes as salves, it is vital to administer them as soon as possible while the wound is still open.

ENZYME SUPPLEMENTATION SUGGESTIONS:

Bee sting

High Amylase Formula: open capsule and mix with a very small amount of tepid water. Apply to the sting and reapply after five minutes.

High Amylase Formula three times between meals

Purpose: To overcome symptoms of allergies and for the proper digestion of carbohydrates, especially grains, raw vegetables, and legumes

Each serving should contain approximately:

Amylase blend	22,000 DU	Cellulase blend	400 CU
Glucoamylase	30 AGU	Lactase	300 LacU
Alpha-galactosidase	1,000 GALU	Maltase	300 DP
Protease blend	15,000 HUT	Pectinase	20 endo-PG
Lipase blend	150 FCCFIP		

High Protease Formula three times daily between meals

Purpose: To help support immune function and assist in removing viruses, fungal forms, toxins, bacteria, and heavy metals
Each capsule should contain approximately:

Protease blend	150,000 HUT	Serratiopeptidase	25,000 units
Mucolase	8 mg	Nattokinase blend	400 FU
Catalase	50 baker units		

Wasp sting

High Protease Formula: open capsule and mix with a very small amount of tepid water. Apply to the sting and reapply after five minutes.
High Protease Formula three times daily between meals
(See above for High Protease Formula specifics)

Spider bite

High Protease Formula: open capsule and mix with a very small amount of tepid water. Apply to the sting and reapply after five minutes. The anti-inflammatory formula is even better when applied to the bite.
High Protease Formula three times daily between meals
(See above for High Protease Formula specifics)

INSOMNIA

Insomnia is defined as habitual sleeplessness, repeated night after night. Most individuals suffering from this ailment have difficulty falling asleep or staying asleep. Although commonly thought of as a sleep disorder, insomnia is typically a symptom of some other problem or disorder. Half of insomnia cases result from excessive worry, stress, an overactive mind, or physical pain. Insomnia can also result from certain drugs, hypoglycemia, asthma, fear, indigestion, poor diet, caffeine, or a deficiency of certain nutrients, including calcium, potassium, and magnesium.

Symptoms associated with insomnia include daytime fatigue, irritability, lack of focus, and difficulty coping with complex tasks. To reduce the instance of insomnia, recommendations include reducing stress levels, getting regular exercise, eating a healthy diet, reducing caffeine and alcohol intake, and maintaining a regular schedule. Enzymes can be used to improve digestion and nutrient uptake and support the health and balance of the body's systems.

ENZYME SUPPLEMENTATION SUGGESTIONS:

*High Potency Digestive Formula with every meal

Purpose: To radically enhance the digestion and assimilation of food while reducing the body's need to produce digestive enzymes; the higher potency formula will average about three times the potency of the average digestive formula; an average formula may be substituted if three times the regular dose is taken

Each serving should contain approximately:

Amylase blend	22,000 DU	Alpha-galactosidase	450 GALU
Protease blend	80,000 HUT	Phytase	50 PU
Lipase blend	3,000 FCCFIP	Pectinase	50 AJDU
Cellulase blend	2,000 CU	Xylanase	500 XU
Invertase	80 IAU	Hemicellulase	30 HCU
Lactase	900 LacU	Beta-glucanase	25 BGU
Maltase	200 DP	L. acidophilus	250 million CFU
Glucoamylase	50 AGU		

*pH Balancing Formula two times daily, morning and night

Purpose: To help the body achieve an optimal pH

Each serving should contain approximately:

Amylase blend	25,000 DU	Lipase blend	175 FCCFIP
Cellulase blend	6,000 CU	Pectinase/Phytase	200 PU
Mineral blend	Potassium bicarbonate, sodium bicarbonate, magnesium citrate	Herbal blend	Hydrilla, marshmallow, papaya
Protease blend	1,000 HUT		

The formula should not exceed 8.0 on the pH scale and the capsule should be enteric coated.

High Protease Formula two times daily, morning and night

Purpose: To help support immune function and assist in removing viruses, fungal forms, toxins, bacteria, and heavy metals

Each capsule should contain approximately:

Protease blend	150,000 HUT	Serratiopeptidase	25,000 units
Mucolase	8 mg	Nattokinase blend	400 FU
Catalase	50 baker units		

IRRITABLE BOWEL SYNDROME

Irritable bowel syndrome (IBS; often called irritable colon or spastic colon) is a disturbance of involuntary muscle movement in the large intestine. IBS is a functional bowel disorder characterized by abdominal pain and changes in bowel habits not associated with any abnormalities. The cause of this ailment is not fully understood.

Symptoms include intermittent abdominal pain and irregular bowel habits (constipation, diarrhea, or both). Long-term IBS can contribute to enzyme and nutrient deficiencies, which in turn can compromise the immune system and interfere with the body's energy production.

Recommendations include dietary changes (including removing starches, high-fat foods, and fried foods); getting regular exercise; eating smaller meals; identifying and avoiding food allergens, particularly gluten (see CELIAC DISEASE); and reducing stress. Enzyme therapy can be used to improve digestion and nutrient absorption and soothe the digestive tract, and probiotics can help maintain the balance of flora in the intestines.

ENZYME SUPPLEMENTATION SUGGESTIONS:

*High Potency Digestive Formula with every meal

Purpose: To radically enhance the digestion and assimilation of food while reducing the body's need to produce digestive enzymes; the higher potency formula will average about three times the potency of the average digestive formula; an average formula may be substituted if three times the regular dose is taken
Each serving should contain approximately:

Amylase blend	22,000 DU	Alpha-galactosidase	450 GALU
Protease blend	80,000 HUT	Phytase	50 PU
Lipase blend	3,000 FCCFIP	Pectinase	50 AJDU
Cellulase blend	2,000 CU	Xylanase	500 XU
Invertase	80 IAU	Hemicellulase	30 HCU
Lactase	900 LacU	Beta-glucanase	25 BGU
Maltase	200 DP	L. acidophilus	250 million CFU
Glucoamylase	50 AGU		

*Soothing Digestive Formula after every meal and anytime there is discomfort

Purpose: To help alleviate conditions associated with gastrointestinal distress

Each serving should contain approximately:

Amylase blend	2,000 DU	Gotu kola	50 mg
Lipase blend	175 FCCFIP	Papaya leaf	100 mg
Cellulase blend	400 CU	Prickly ash bark	50 mg
Marshmallow root	100 mg		

Additional helpful ingredients:

DGL (deglycyrrhizinated licorice)	

This formula should *not* contain protease. Other herbs may also be present.

*Probiotic Formula daily

Purpose: To assist the body in balancing microflora
Each serving should contain approximately 5 billion probiotic live cells (guaranteed potency), comprised of:

Bacillus Subtillis	No less than 3 billion CFU guaranteed potency	A blend of *L. acidophilus, L. casei, L. bulgaris, L. plantarum, L. rhamnosus, L. salivarius*	No less than 1 billion CFU guaranteed potency
L. paracassei F-19	No less than 1 billion CFU guaranteed potency		

JOINT PAIN

See ARTHRITIS.

JOCK ITCH

See RINGWORM.

KIDNEY STRESS

The kidneys are the organs responsible for filtering the blood and removing waste products, sodium, and excess water, which are released from the kidneys in the form of urine into the bladder. The most important waste products for the kidneys to eliminate are those generated by the breakdown of proteins, which control the body's acid balance. In that way, the kidneys regulate pH balance. These organs also regulate mineral ion concentration (particularly potassium), produce hormones that affect red blood cell production, and convert vitamin D into an active hormonal form. Overall, the health of the kidneys directly affects the health of the entire body.

Kidney imbalances can result from genetic disorders, xenobiotics (including heavy metal toxicity), kidney stones, and bacterial infections. Enzymes can help support overall kidney health by improving digestion and nutrient absorption, strengthening the immune system, aiding the process of balancing pH levels, and reducing inflammation of the kidneys during times of distress or illness.

IMPORTANT NOTE: If you are experiencing back pain in your midback, frequent urination or difficulty urinating, or burning or abdominal pain when you urinate, you should immediately seek medical attention.

ENZYME SUPPLEMENTATION SUGGESTIONS:

*High Potency Digestive Formula with every meal

Purpose: To radically enhance the digestion and assimilation of food while reducing the body's need to produce digestive enzymes; the higher potency formula will average about three times the potency of the average digestive formula; an average formula may be substituted if three times the regular dose is taken

Each serving should contain approximately:

Amylase blend	22,000 DU	Alpha-galactosidase	450 GALU
Protease blend	80,000 HUT	Phytase	50 PU
Lipase blend	3,000 FCCFIP	Pectinase	50 AJDU
Cellulase blend	2,000 CU	Xylanase	500 XU
Invertase	80 IAU	Hemicellulase	30 HCU
Lactase	900 LacU	Beta-glucanase	25 BGU
Maltase	200 DP	L. acidophilus	250 million CFU
Glucoamylase	50 AGU		

*High Protease Formula three to four times daily

Purpose: To help support immune function and assist in removing viruses, fungal forms, toxins, bacteria, and heavy metals

Each capsule should contain approximately:

Protease blend	150,000 HUT	Serratiopeptidase	25,000 units
Mucolase	8 mg	Nattokinase blend	400 FU
Catalase	50 baker units		

*pH Balancing Formula three times daily

Purpose: To help the body achieve an optimal pH
Each serving should contain approximately:

Amylase blend	25,000 DU	Lipase blend	175 FCCFIP
Cellulase blend	6,000 CU	Pectinase/Phytase	200 PU
Mineral blend	Potassium bicarbonate, sodium bicarbonate, magnesium citrate	Herbal blend	Hydrilla, marshmallow, papaya
Protease blend	1,000 HUT		

The formula should not exceed 8.0 on the pH scale and the capsule should be enteric coated.

Anti-inflammatory Formula may be added for inflammation or pain

Purpose: To address inflammation, speed recovery, and repair tissue; best if enteric coated
Each serving should contain approximately:

Protease blend	120,000 HUT	Amylase blend	7,000 DU
Papain	140,000 PU	Lipase blend	600 FCCFIP
Bromelain	1,200 GDU (11.25 million FCCPU)	Catalase	100 baker units

LACTOSE INTOLERANCE

A deficiency in lactase, the enzyme responsible for digesting the lactose present in dairy products, is common throughout the world. Lactase breaks lactose, or milk sugar, down into simple sugars to be absorbed by the body. When lactase is deficient, lactose sits in the colon undigested and ferments, causing FLATULENCE, cramping, bloating, watery diarrhea, and possibly nausea.

Lactase deficiency is more common in some ethnic groups (black, Asian, Hispanic) than in others. Most people are born with the ability to produce lactase but many lose the ability with age. Many children lose the ability to produce lactase by three to seven years of age.

Recommendations include avoiding or limiting the intake of dairy products, taking digestive enzymes with meals, and supplementing with probiotics to promote recolonization of the gastrointestinal tract.

ENZYME SUPPLEMENTATION SUGGESTIONS:

*Dairy Digesting Formula or High Potency Digestive Formula with every meal

Purpose: To help break down the common allergens in dairy, which includes lactose and casein
    Each serving should contain approximately:

Lactase	9,000 ALU	Amylase blend	7,500 DU
Protease blend	25,000 HUT	Glucoamylase	25 AG
Lipase blend	500 FCCFIP	Malstase	350 DP
Cellulase	300 CU		

*Probiotic Formula daily before bed

Purpose: To assist the body in balancing microflora
    Each serving should contain approximately 5 billion probiotic live cells (guaranteed potency), comprised of:

Bacillus Subtillis	No less than 3 billion CFU guaranteed potency	A blend of *L. acidophilus, L. casei, L. bulgaris, L. plantarum, L. rhamnosus, L. salivarius*	No less than 1 billion CFU guaranteed potency
L. paracassei F-19	No less than 1 billion CFU guaranteed potency		

High Potency Digestive Formula with every meal
Purpose: To radically enhance the digestion and assimilation of food while reducing the body's need to produce digestive enzymes; the higher potency formula will average about three times the potency of the average digestive formula; an average formula may be substituted if three times the regular dose is taken
    Each serving should contain approximately:

Amylase blend	22,000 DU	Alpha-galactosidase	450 GALU
Protease blend	80,000 HUT	Phytase	50 PU
Lipase blend	3,000 FCCFIP	Pectinase	50 AJDU
Cellulase blend	2,000 CU	Xylanase	500 XU
Invertase	80 IAU	Hemicellulase	30 HCU
Lactase	900 LacU	Beta-glucanase	25 BGU
Maltase	200 DP	*L. acidophilus*	250 million CFU
Glucoamylase	50 AGU		

LARYNGITIS

Laryngitis is an inflammation of the mucous membranes of the larynx and irritation of the vocal chords. Laryngitis is characterized by dryness and soreness of the throat, hoarseness, coughing, and impaired speech. Often caused by a virus or bacteria, it may also be aggravated by smoking, allergic reactions, reflux, and straining the voice.

Recommendations include ascertaining the underlying cause of the laryngitis, increasing hydration, rest, and supporting the immune system. Enzymes can also be used to improve digestion, soothe the digestive tract, and reduce inflammation.

ENZYME SUPPLEMENTATION SUGGESTIONS:
*High Protease Formula three times a day on an empty stomach

Purpose: To help support immune function and assist in removing viruses, fungal forms, toxins, bacteria, and heavy metals
Each capsule should contain approximately:

Protease blend	150,000 HUT	Serratiopeptidase	25,000 units
Mucolase	8 mg	Nattokinase blend	400 FU
Catalase	50 baker units		

*Anti-inflammatory Formula may be taken anytime for inflammation

Purpose: To address inflammation, speed recovery, and repair tissue; best if enteric coated
Each serving should contain approximately:

Protease blend	120,000 HUT	Amylase blend	7,000 DU
Papain	140,000 PU	Lipase blend	600 FCCFIP
Bromelain	1,200 GDU (11.25 million FCCPU)	Catalase	100 baker units

High Potency Digestive Formula with every meal

Purpose: To radically enhance the digestion and assimilation of food while reducing the body's need to produce digestive enzymes; the higher potency formula will average about three times the potency of the average digestive formula; an average formula may be substituted if three times the regular dose is taken

Each serving should contain approximately:

Amylase blend	22,000 DU	Alpha-galactosidase	450 GALU
Protease blend	80,000 HUT	Phytase	50 PU
Lipase blend	3,000 FCCFIP	Pectinase	50 AJDU
Cellulase blend	2,000 CU	Xylanase	500 XU
Invertase	80 IAU	Hemicellulase	30 HCU
Lactase	900 LacU	Beta-glucanase	25 BGU
Maltase	200 DP	L. acidophilus	250 million CFU
Glucoamylase	50 AGU		

Soothing Digestive Formula: open capsules, mix with water, and drink

Purpose: To help alleviate conditions associated with gastrointestinal distress
Each serving should contain approximately:

Amylase blend	2,000 DU	Gotu kola	50 mg
Lipase blend	175 FCCFIP	Papaya leaf	100 mg
Cellulase blend	400 CU	Prickly ash bark	50 mg
Marshmallow root	100 mg		

Additional helpful ingredients:

DGL (deglycyrrhizinated licorice)	

This formula should *not* contain protease. Other herbs may also be present.

LIVER TOXICITY

The liver is the largest gland in the body and the second largest organ. Located immediately beneath the right side of the diaphragm, it weighs nearly four pounds. This gland has many vital functions and plays a major role in metabolism, in eliminating toxins from the body, and in storing nutrients. The liver produces bile that aids in the digestion of fats, produces proteins for blood plasma, and produces cholesterol and special proteins that help to carry fats around the body. The liver also stores glycogen and filters out drugs and poisonous substances that would otherwise accumulate in the bloodstream.

The liver is extremely resilient. Up to 75 percent of its cells can be destroyed or surgically removed before it ceases to function. The most common cause of liver disease in the United States is alcohol consumption. Hepatitis is also a common liver disease.

Considering the important role the liver plays in our bodies, it is critical to keep it healthy and functioning. Enzymes can be used to support liver health by improving digestion and nutrient absorption, managing the digestion of fats, strengthening the immune system, and reducing inflammation if the liver is under attack during illness.

ENZYME SUPPLEMENTATION SUGGESTIONS:

*High Potency Digestive Formula and/or High Lipase Formula with every meal

Purpose: To radically enhance the digestion and assimilation of food while reducing the body's need to produce digestive enzymes; the higher potency formula will average about three times the potency of the average digestive formula; an average formula may be substituted if three times the regular dose is taken
Each serving should contain approximately:

Amylase blend	22,000 DU	Alpha-galactosidase	450 GALU
Protease blend	80,000 HUT	Phytase	50 PU
Lipase blend	3,000 FCCFIP	Pectinase	50 AJDU
Cellulase blend	2,000 CU	Xylanase	500 XU
Invertase	80 IAU	Hemicellulase	30 HCU
Lactase	900 LacU	Beta-glucanase	25 BGU
Maltase	200 DP	L. acidophilus	250 million CFU
Glucoamylase	50 AGU		

*High Lipase Formula three times daily between meals

Purpose: To improve fat digestion and metabolism, and reduce stress to the liver
Each capsule should contain approximately:

Lipase blend	5,000 FCCFIP	Protease blend	20,000 HUT
Amylase blend	10,000 DU	Lactase	300 LacU

*High Protease Formula four times daily between meals

Purpose: To help support immune function and assist in removing viruses, fungal forms, toxins, bacteria, and heavy metals
Each capsule should contain approximately:

Protease blend	150,000 HUT	Serratiopeptidase	25,000 units
Mucolase	8 mg	Nattokinase blend	400 FU
Catalase	50 baker units		

Anti-inflammatory Formula may be added for inflammation

Purpose: To address inflammation, speed recovery, and repair tissue; best if enteric coated

　　Each serving should contain approximately:

Protease blend	120,000 HUT	Amylase blend	7,000 DU
Papain	140,000 PU	Lipase blend	600 FCCFIP
Bromelain	1,200 GDU (11.25 million FCCPU)	Catalase	100 baker units

LONGEVITY

Longevity is the length of a person's life. Research has produced many different theories of the aging process. (See also AGING.) Two predominant theories of aging are the damage theory and the programmed theory. The damage theory advocates that the aging process is a result of cumulative damage to genetic materials and cells. The programmed theory states that old age is determined by a clocklike genetic mechanism in the body. Although there are no magic cures to arrest the aging process, there are measures that one can take to slow the process and reduce the risks of premature death.

　　Significant factors that may contribute to an individual's longevity include genetics, access to health care, hygiene, diet, exercise, and lifestyle. Therefore, recommendations to increase longevity include a healthy, well-balanced diet, stress management, rest, regular exercise, support of the digestive and immune systems, and enzyme supplementation for overall improved health.

ENZYME SUPPLEMENTATION SUGGESTIONS:

*High Potency Digestive Formula with every meal

Purpose: To radically enhance the digestion and assimilation of food while reducing the body's need to produce digestive enzymes; the higher potency formula will average about three times the potency of the average digestive formula; an average formula may be substituted if three times the regular dose is taken

　　Each serving should contain approximately:

Amylase blend	22,000 DU	Alpha-galactosidase	450 GALU
Protease blend	80,000 HUT	Phytase	50 PU
Lipase blend	3,000 FCCFIP	Pectinase	50 AJDU
Cellulase blend	2,000 CU	Xylanase	500 XU
Invertase	80 IAU	Hemicellulase	30 HCU
Lactase	900 LacU	Beta-glucanase	25 BGU
Maltase	200 DP	*L. acidophilus*	250 million CFU
Glucoamylase	50 AGU		

*High Protease Formula three times per day

Purpose: To help support immune function and assist in removing viruses, fungal forms, toxins, bacteria, and heavy metals
Each capsule should contain approximately:

Protease blend	150,000 HUT	Serratiopeptidase	25,000 units
Mucolase	8 mg	Nattokinase blend	400 FU
Catalase	50 baker units		

*Nattokinase Formula two times per day

Purpose: To support cardiovascular health and decrease blood pressure by breaking down fibrin
Each serving should contain approximately:
Necessary ingredient:

Nattokinase NSK-SD	1,000 FU

Helpful ingredients:

Amylase blend	9,000 DU	Glucoamylase	25 AGU
Protease blend	20,000 HUT	Lipase blend	1,000 FCCFIP
Minerals	85 mg	Cellulase blend	400 CU

*pH Balancing Formula two times per day, morning and night

Purpose: To help the body achieve an optimal pH
Each serving should contain approximately:

Amylase blend	25,000 DU	Lipase blend	175 FCCFIP
Cellulase blend	6,000 CU	Pectinase/Phytase	200 PU
Mineral blend	Potassium bicarbonate, sodium bicarbonate, magnesium citrate	Herbal blend	Hydrilla, marshmallow, papaya
Protease blend	1,000 HUT		

The formula should not exceed 8.0 on the pH scale and the capsule should be enteric coated.

LUPUS

Lupus is a chronic, inflammatory autoimmune disease in which the body's immune system attacks itself. The specific cause of this disorder has not yet been ascertained; however, many researchers believe that it may be triggered by a virus.

Approximately 90 percent of individuals diagnosed with lupus are female; the disease most often arises in women between the ages of fifteen and forty-five.

There are two different forms of lupus. Discoid lupus erythematosus affects the skin. A butterfly-shape rash forms over the cheeks and nose; it typically flares up with sun exposure. Additional symptoms of this skin disease include small, soft groups of lesions that appear on the skin, producing scarring. The second form of lupus is systemic lupus erythematosus, which affects the organs, blood vessels, and joints of the body. Many individuals afflicted with systemic lupus erythematosus develop nephritis, or inflammation of the kidneys, which can lead to more serious kidney and health problems.

The symptoms of lupus vary depending upon the condition and the antibodies the immune system produces. The most common symptoms are achy joints, inflammation of the joints, fever, fatigue, weakness, hair loss, anemia, abnormal blood clotting, and mouth or nose ulcers.

Both types of lupus periodically flare up and then go into remission. Infections, childbirth, excessive stress, fatigue, certain chemicals, and drugs can precipitate attacks. Serious cases of lupus can adversely affect the kidneys, heart, nervous system, and brain, resulting in psychosis, depression, seizures, and amnesia.

Recommendations include avoiding prolonged exposure to sunlight, lifestyle modification to reduce stress, promoting sufficient rest and sleep, and dietary changes to lower fat and salt intake, as well as enzyme supplementation to support the kidneys, digestive system, and immune system. Enzymes can also be used to treat inflammation and balance the pH levels to support overall health.

ENZYME SUPPLEMENTATION SUGGESTIONS:

*High Potency Digestive Formula with meals

Purpose: To radically enhance the digestion and assimilation of food while reducing the body's need to produce digestive enzymes; the higher potency formula will average about three times the potency of the average digestive formula; an average formula may be substituted if three times the regular dose is taken

Each serving should contain approximately:

Amylase blend	22,000 DU	Alpha-galactosidase	450 GALU
Protease blend	80,000 HUT	Phytase	50 PU
Lipase blend	3,000 FCCFIP	Pectinase	50 AJDU
Cellulase blend	2,000 CU	Xylanase	500 XU
Invertase	80 IAU	Hemicellulase	30 HCU
Lactase	900 LacU	Beta-glucanase	25 BGU
Maltase	200 DP	L. acidophilus	250 million CFU
Glucoamylase	50 AGU		

*Anti-inflammatory Formula three to four times daily

Purpose: To address inflammation, speed recovery, and repair tissue; best if enteric coated

Each serving should contain approximately:

Protease blend	120,000 HUT	Amylase blend	7,000 DU
Papain	140,000 PU	Lipase blend	600 FCCFIP
Bromelain	1,200 GDU (11.25 million FCCPU)	Catalase	100 baker units

*pH Balancing Formula three times daily

Purpose: To help the body achieve an optimal pH

Each serving should contain approximately:

Amylase blend	25,000 DU	Lipase blend	175 FCCFIP
Cellulase blend	6,000 CU	Pectinase/Phytase	200 PU
Mineral blend	Potassium bicarbonate, sodium bicarbonate, magnesium citrate	Herbal blend	Hydrilla, marshmallow, papaya
Protease blend	1,000 HUT		

The formula should not exceed 8.0 on the pH scale and the capsule should be enteric coated.

Serratiopeptidase Formula may be added to the anti-inflammatory formula for chronic pain

Purpose: To break down protein and reduce inflammation. Also supports cardiovascular health and enhances other proteases.

Each serving should contain approximately:

Serratiopeptidase	80,000 SU
Protease blend	70,000 HUT
Mineral blend	50 mg

Supporting enzymes:

Bromelain	Papain

High Protease Formula three to four times daily

Purpose: To help support immune function and assist in removing viruses, fungal forms, toxins, bacteria, and heavy metals

Each capsule should contain approximately:

Protease blend	150,000 HUT	Serratiopeptidase	25,000 units
Mucolase	8 mg	Nattokinase blend	400 FU
Catalase	50 baker units		

LYME DISEASE

Lyme disease is the result of a deer tick bite and is caused by infection from *Borrelia burgdorferi* bacteria. Sometimes it is misdiagnosed as multiple sclerosis, rheumatoid arthritis, fibromyalgia, chronic fatigue syndrome, or other (mainly autoimmune and neurological) diseases. Lyme disease is considered one of the fastest growing infectious diseases in the United States.

The first symptom of this condition is generally the appearance of a rash and a red papule on the skin a few days following a tick bite. Acute (early) reactions can include flulike symptoms, including fever, fatigue, malaise, a stiff neck, backache, headache, joint pain and swelling, sinus infection, heart palpitations, nausea and vomiting. Chronic (late) symptoms may include muscle twitching, seizures, panic attacks, depression, hallucinations, and adrenal disorders. Left undetected, Lyme disease can cause spleen and lymph node enlargement, arthritis, brain damage, and an irregular heart rhythm. Symptoms usually subside slowly over a period of two to three years.

Although antibiotic therapies are generally implemented, no cure has yet been found. If Lyme disease is suspected, consult with a physician as soon as possible. The sooner antibiotics are used, the more successful they are. Enzymes can be used to support proper functioning of the immune and digestive systems, to reduce inflammation and pain, and to balance the pH levels in the body to promote overall health.

ENZYME SUPPLEMENTATION SUGGESTIONS:

*High Potency Digestive Formula with every meal

Purpose: To radically enhance the digestion and assimilation of food while reducing the body's need to produce digestive enzymes; the higher potency formula will average about three times the potency of the average digestive formula; an average formula may be substituted if three times the regular dose is taken

Each serving should contain approximately:

Amylase blend	22,000 DU	Alpha-galactosidase	450 GALU
Protease blend	80,000 HUT	Phytase	50 PU
Lipase blend	3,000 FCCFIP	Pectinase	50 AJDU
Cellulase blend	2,000 CU	Xylanase	500 XU
Invertase	80 IAU	Hemicellulase	30 HCU
Lactase	900 LacU	Beta-glucanase	25 BGU
Maltase	200 DP	L. acidophilus	250 million CFU
Glucoamylase	50 AGU		

*High Protease Formula three times daily between meals

Purpose: To help support immune function and assist in removing viruses, fungal forms, toxins, bacteria, and heavy metals

Each capsule should contain approximately:

Protease blend	150,000 HUT	Serratiopeptidase	25,000 units
Mucolase	8 mg	Nattokinase blend	400 FU
Catalase	50 baker units		

Serratiopeptidase Formula

Purpose: To break down protein and reduce inflammation. Also supports cardiovascular health and enhances other proteases.

Each serving should contain approximately:

Serratiopeptidase	80,000 SU
Protease blend	70,000 HUT
Mineral blend	50 mg

Supporting enzymes:

Bromelain	Papain

Anti-inflammatory Formula three times daily or whenever needed

Purpose: To address inflammation, speed recovery, and repair tissue; best if enteric coated

Each serving should contain approximately:

Protease blend	120,000 HUT	Amylase blend	7,000 DU
Papain	140,000 PU	Lipase blend	600 FCCFIP
Bromelain	1,200 GDU (11.25 million FCCPU)	Catalase	100 baker units

Optional: pH Balancing Formula three times daily

Purpose: To help the body achieve an optimal pH

Each serving should contain approximately:

Amylase blend	25,000 DU	Lipase blend	175 FCCFIP
Cellulase blend	6,000 CU	Pectinase/Phytase	200 PU
Mineral blend	Potassium bicarbonate, sodium bicarbonate, magnesium citrate	Herbal blend	Hydrilla, marshmallow, papaya
Protease blend	1,000 HUT		

The formula should not exceed 8.0 on the pH scale and the capsule should be enteric coated.

LYMPHATIC CONGESTION

The lymphatic system, a major component of the immune system, is a network of fluids, organs, and vessels. The primary parts of the lymph system include the lymph nodes, spleen, appendix, tonsils, adenoids, and Peyer's patch in the small intestine. Their functions include the transportation of fatty acids from the small intestine to important locations throughout the body, the defense of the body against aggressive agents (pathogens such as bacteria, viruses, and toxins), and the destruction of accumulated wastes or cellular debris. See chapter 3 and appendix C for more information on the functioning of the immune system.

All body tissues are bathed in a watery fluid derived from the bloodstream called lymph. There are approximately six to ten liters of lymph fluids in the body, which is approximately two times the amount of blood. The fluid is transported through the body in lymphatic vessels similar to blood vessels. These vessels connect with the capillaries so that lymph fluid can be absorbed into and out of the bloodstream. The lymph system does not contain a pump like the heart, so circulation of the lymph fluid occurs as a result of contraction of the muscles throughout the body.

The flow of lymph fluid can stagnate from dehydration, fatigue, infection, stress, or a lack of physical activity. This may result in lymphostatic edema, and as toxins accumulate various metabolic problems or infections may occur. One of the best ways to support lymphatic circulation and reduce lymphatic congestion is to increase physical activity. Enzymes can be used to improve digestion, support the immune system, improve absorption of critical fatty acids, and reduce inflammation that may occur in the elements of the lymphatic system.

ENZYME SUPPLEMENTATION SUGGESTIONS:

*High Potency Digestive Formula with every meal

Purpose: To radically enhance the digestion and assimilation of food while reducing the body's need to produce digestive enzymes; the higher potency formula will average about three times the potency of the average digestive formula; an average formula may be substituted if three times the regular dose is taken
Each serving should contain approximately:

Amylase blend	22,000 DU	Alpha-galactosidase	450 GALU
Protease blend	80,000 HUT	Phytase	50 PU
Lipase blend	3,000 FCCFIP	Pectinase	50 AJDU
Cellulase blend	2,000 CU	Xylanase	500 XU
Invertase	80 IAU	Hemicellulase	30 HCU
Lactase	900 LacU	Beta-glucanase	25 BGU
Maltase	200 DP	L. acidophilus	250 million CFU
Glucoamylase	50 AGU		

*High Protease Formula three times daily

Purpose: To help support immune function and assist in removing viruses, fungal forms, toxins, bacteria, and heavy metals
Each capsule should contain approximately:

Protease blend	150,000 HUT	Serratiopeptidase	25,000 units
Mucolase	8 mg	Nattokinase blend	400 FU
Catalase	50 baker units		

High Lipase Formula three times daily

Purpose: To improve fat digestion and metabolism, as well as the health of the cardiovascular system

Each capsule should contain approximately:

Lipase blend	5,000 FCCFIP	Protease blend	20,000 HUT
Amylase blend	10,000 DU	Lactase	300 LacU

Anti-inflammatory Formula as needed for inflammation

Purpose: To address inflammation, speed recovery, and repair tissue; best if enteric coated

Each serving should contain approximately:

Protease blend	120,000 HUT	Amylase blend	7,000 DU
Papain	140,000 PU	Lipase blend	600 FCCFIP
Bromelain	1,200 GDU (11.25 million FCCPU)	Catalase	100 baker units

MALABSORPTION SYNDROME

Malabsorption syndrome is a change in the body's ability to absorb nutrients into the bloodstream from the intestines. This imbalance typically involves impaired absorption of nutrients, vitamins, and minerals in the lining of the small intestine. If the intestinal tract mucosa lining is impaired or there is some blockage to the flow of digested foods, then absorption becomes a problem. Without the absorption of key nutrients, a domino effect can occur in the system and take many different forms of ill health. Therefore, cleansing and support of the intestinal tract and mucosa lining is imperative.

Malabsorption syndrome can exist without an underlying cause, but it is often associated with other disorders, such as CYSTIC FIBROSIS, CELIAC DISEASE, chronic pancreatitis, LACTOSE INTOLERANCE, and GLUTEN INTOLERANCE (sprue, Crohn's disease; see INFLAMMATORY BOWEL DISEASE).

The most common symptoms of this syndrome are anemia, diarrhea, bloating, abdominal cramping, edema (fluid retention), weight loss, muscle cramping, fatigue, and weakness.

Enzyme therapies can be helpful in improving digestion and soothing the digestive tract, supporting the immune system, supporting the balance of bacteria in the intestines, and reducing inflammation of the gastrointestinal tract.

ENZYME SUPPLEMENTATION SUGGESTIONS:

*High Potency Digestive Formula with every meal

Purpose: To radically enhance the digestion and assimilation of food while reducing the body's need to produce digestive enzymes; the higher potency formula will average about three times the potency of the average digestive formula; an average formula may be substituted if three times the regular dose is taken

Each serving should contain approximately:

Amylase blend	22,000 DU	Alpha-galactosidase	450 GALU
Protease blend	80,000 HUT	Phytase	50 PU
Lipase blend	3,000 FCCFIP	Pectinase	50 AJDU
Cellulase blend	2,000 CU	Xylanase	500 XU
Invertase	80 IAU	Hemicellulase	30 HCU
Lactase	900 LacU	Beta-glucanase	25 BGU
Maltase	200 DP	L. acidophilus	250 million CFU
Glucoamylase	50 AGU		

*Probiotic Formula daily before bed

Purpose: To assist the body in balancing microflora

Each serving should contain approximately 5 billion probiotic live cells (guaranteed potency), comprised of:

Bacillus Subtillis	No less than 3 billion CFU guaranteed potency	A blend of L. acidophilus, L. casei, L. bulgaris, L. plantarum, L. rhamnosus, L. salivarius	No less than 1 billion CFU guaranteed potency
L. paracassei F-19	No less than 1 billion CFU guaranteed potency		

High Cellulase Formula three times daily for one to two weeks

Purpose: To manage yeast overgrowth

Each capsule should contain approximately:

Cellulase blend	30,000 CU
Protease blend	100,000 HUT

Contraindications: High amounts of cellulase should not be taken with certain timed-release medications that contain cellulose.

Soothing Digestive Formula three times daily (to help rebuild mucosal lining)

Purpose: To help alleviate conditions associated with gastrointestinal distress

Each serving should contain approximately:

Amylase blend	2,000 DU	Gotu kola	50 mg
Lipase blend	175 FCCFIP	Papaya leaf	100 mg
Cellulase blend	400 CU	Prickly ash bark	50 mg
Marshmallow root	100 mg		

Additional helpful ingredients:

DGL (deglycyrrhizinated licorice)	

This formula should *not* contain protease. Other herbs may also be present.

High Protease Formula or **Anti-inflammatory Formula** may be added as needed

Purpose: To help support immune function and assist in removing viruses, fungal forms, toxins, bacteria, and heavy metals

Each capsule should contain approximately:

Protease blend	150,000 HUT	Serratiopeptidase	25,000 units
Mucolase	8 mg	Nattokinase blend	400 FU
Catalase	50 baker units		

Purpose: To address inflammation, speed recovery, and repair tissue; best if enteric coated

Each serving should contain approximately:

Protease blend	120,000 HUT	Amylase blend	7,000 DU
Papain	140,000 PU	Lipase blend	600 FCCFIP
Bromelain	1,200 GDU (11.25 million FCCPU)	Catalase	100 baker units

MENOPAUSE

Menopause occurs as the ovaries stop producing estrogen, causing the reproductive system to gradually stop functioning. Technically, menopause refers to the cessation of menstruation (ovulation), as a natural part of a woman's normal aging process. It is a time in a woman's life when physical and psychological changes occur. The average age at the onset of menopause is fifty years.

The most common symptoms or side effects of menopause include hot flashes and night sweats, occurring in approximately 70 percent of all menopausal women. Additional symptoms may include headaches, atrophic vaginitis, frequent urinary tract infections, forgetfulness, and cold hands and feet (poor circulation). These symptoms occur as a result of changing hormone levels in the body and the body's attempt to balance those hormone levels.

Psychological symptoms are often attributed to menopause, but it is not clear whether these symptoms are caused by the lack of estrogen or are a reaction to the physical symptoms and the sleep disturbances caused by the night sweats. The most common nonphysical symptoms are poor memory, poor concentration, tearfulness, anxiety, and loss of interest in sex.

Changes in metabolism (internal chemistry) also occur during menopause, but may not cause symptoms until later. The bones lose calcium more rapidly, especially in the first two to five years of the period. Other metabolic effects include a possible rise in blood pressure and an increase in fats in the blood.

A common remedy offered for some of the symptoms is estrogen replacement therapy. Because estrogen is associated with side effects and long-term risks as well as benefits, a woman and her doctor must weigh the benefits against the risks before deciding whether to use estrogen replacement therapy. Side effects of estrogen therapy may include nausea, breast discomfort, headaches, and mood swings. The possibility that estrogen might increase the risk of breast cancer has long been a concern. For women who are already at high risk, it is not recommended. Postmenopausal women who take estrogen without progesterone have an increased risk of endometrial cancer (cancer of the lining of the uterus). The risk of developing gallbladder disease is modestly increased during the first year of estrogen replacement therapy.

Premature menopause occurs before the age of 40. Possible causes include a genetic predisposition and autoimmune disorders, in which antibodies are produced that can damage a number of glands, including the ovaries. Smoking has also been known to cause early menopause.

Artificial menopause results from medical intervention that reduces or stops hormone secretion by the ovaries. These interventions include surgery to remove the ovaries or reduce their blood supply, and chemotherapy or radiation therapy to the pelvis to treat cancer. Surgery to remove the uterus (hysterectomy) ends menstrual periods, but it does not affect hormone levels as long as the ovaries are intact, and therefore should not cause menopause.

Nutritional needs become an important focus for menopausal women. The changes in the body's metabolic capability, hormonal structure, and digestive capabilities, like the aging factor, cannot be stopped, but can be addressed to support the optimal nutritional potential available to keep a woman at peak health.

Recommendations include a well-balanced diet, stress management, rest, regular exercise, and glandular/hormonal support. Enzyme therapy can support the digestive and immune systems, improve the digestion of fats, improve pH balance, and treat any inflammation that may occur as a side effect.

ENZYME SUPPLEMENTATION SUGGESTIONS:

*High Potency Digestive Formula with every meal

Purpose: To radically enhance the digestion and assimilation of food while reducing the body's need to produce digestive enzymes; the higher potency formula will average about three times the potency of the average digestive formula; an average formula may be substituted if three times the regular dose is taken

Each serving should contain approximately:

Amylase blend	22,000 DU	Alpha-galactosidase	450 GALU
Protease blend	80,000 HUT	Phytase	50 PU
Lipase blend	3,000 FCCFIP	Pectinase	50 AJDU
Cellulase blend	2,000 CU	Xylanase	500 XU
Invertase	80 IAU	Hemicellulase	30 HCU
Lactase	900 LacU	Beta-glucanase	25 BGU
Maltase	200 DP	L. acidophilus	250 million CFU
Glucoamylase	50 AGU		

*High Lipase Formula three times daily

Purpose: To improve fat digestion and metabolism, as well as support the endocrine system, which produces hormones

Each capsule should contain approximately:

Lipase blend	5,000 FCCFIP	Protease blend	20,000 HUT
Amylase blend	10,000 DU	Lactase	300 LacU

High Protease Formula three times daily

Purpose: To help support immune function and assist in removing viruses, fungal forms, toxins, bacteria, and heavy metals

Each capsule should contain approximately:

Protease blend	150,000 HUT	Serratiopeptidase	25,000 units
Mucolase	8 mg	Nattokinase blend	400 FU
Catalase	50 baker units		

Anti-inflammatory Formula may be added anytime for inflammation

Purpose: To address inflammation, speed recovery, and repair tissue; best if enteric coated

Each serving should contain approximately:

Protease blend	120,000 HUT	Amylase blend	7,000 DU
Papain	140,000 PU	Lipase blend	600 FCCFIP
Bromelain	1,200 GDU (11.25 million FCCPU)	Catalase	100 baker units

MIGRAINES

Migraines are intense and disabling vascular headaches that can last for two hours to two days. Migraines are common, affecting 15 to 20 percent of men and 25 to 30 percent of women. They are characterized by severe pain on one or both sides of the head. They generally involve a throbbing or a pounding sharp pain, and are often accompanied by visual disturbances or nausea and vomiting. In a common migraine, the pain of the headache develops slowly, sometimes mounting to a throbbing pain that is made worse by movement or noise.

Classical migraines are relatively rare. These headaches are preceded by a slowly expanding area of blindness surrounded by a sparkling edge; these symptoms can affect up to one-half of the field of vision of each eye. The blindness may resolve after twenty minutes, and is often followed by a severe one-sided headache with nausea, vomiting, hypersensitivity to light, and hypersensitivity to sound. Other temporary neurological symptoms, such as weakness on one side, may also occur.

Migraine sufferers usually develop their own coping mechanisms for intractable pain. A cold or hot shower directed at the head, a cool wet washcloth, sometimes a warm bath, or resting in a dark and silent room may be as helpful as medication for many patients, but both should be used when needed. A simple treatment that has been effective for some individuals is to place spoonfuls of ice cream on the soft palate at the back of the mouth, to be held with the tongue until they melt. This directs cooling to the hypothalamus, which is suspected to be involved with the migraine feedback cycle, and for some it can stop even a severe headache very quickly.

Causes of migraines include vascular instability, platelet disorders, nerve disorders, seratonin deficiency, certain drugs and xenobiotics, nutrient deficiencies, and allergenic foods.

Recommendations include ascertaining the underlying cause or precipitating factors of the migraines, dietary changes to identify and eliminate food allergies, stress management, adequate rest, and supplementation with enzymes and nutrients that may be deficient in the body. Enzymes can also be used to treat inflammation and to improve circulation when symptoms arise, which may be helpful for some migraine sufferers.

ENZYME SUPPLEMENTATION SUGGESTIONS:

*High Potency Digestive Formula with every meal

Purpose: To radically enhance the digestion and assimilation of food while reducing the body's need to produce digestive enzymes; the higher potency formula will average about three times the potency of the average digestive formula; an average formula may be substituted if three times the regular dose is taken
   Each serving should contain approximately:

Amylase blend	22,000 DU	Alpha-galactosidase	450 GALU
Protease blend	80,000 HUT	Phytase	50 PU
Lipase blend	3,000 FCCFIP	Pectinase	50 AJDU
Cellulase blend	2,000 CU	Xylanase	500 XU
Invertase	80 IAU	Hemicellulase	30 HCU
Lactase	900 LacU	Beta-glucanase	25 BGU
Maltase	200 DP	L. acidophilus	250 million CFU
Glucoamylase	50 AGU		

*Anti-inflammatory Formula anytime symptoms arise

Purpose: To address inflammation, speed recovery, and repair tissue; best if enteric coated
   Each serving should contain approximately:

Protease blend	120,000 HUT	Amylase blend	7,000 DU
Papain	140,000 PU	Lipase blend	600 FCCFIP
Bromelain	1,200 GDU (11.25 million FCCPU)	Catalase	100 baker units

Nattokinase Formula could also be substituted for the anti-inflammatory formula.

Purpose: To support cardiovascular health and decrease blood pressure by breaking down fibrin

Each serving should contain approximately:
Necessary ingredient:

Nattokinase NSK-SD	1,000 FU

Helpful ingredients:

Amylase blend	9,000 DU	Glucoamylase	25 AGU
Protease blend	20,000 HUT	Lipase blend	1,000 FCCFIP
Minerals	85 mg	Cellulase blend	400 CU

Serratiopeptidase Formula could also be substituted for the anti-inflammatory formula.

Purpose: To break down protein and reduce inflammation. Also supports cardiovascular health and enhances other proteases.
Each serving should contain approximately:

Serratiopeptidase	80,000 SU
Protease blend	70,000 HUT
Mineral blend	50 mg

Supporting enzymes:

Bromelain	Papain

High Amylase Formula anytime allergy symptoms arise

Purpose: To overcome symptoms of allergies and for the proper digestion of carbohydrates, especially grains, raw vegetables, and legumes
Each serving should contain approximately:

Amylase blend	22,000 DU	Cellulase blend	400 CU
Glucoamylase	30 AGU	Lactase	300 LacU
Alpha-galactosidase	1,000 GALU	Maltase	300 DP
Protease blend	15,000 HUT	Pectinase	20 endo-PG
Lipase blend	150 FCCFIP		

MUCUS CONGESTION

The mucous membranes in the body are involved in absorption and secretion. They line the various body cavities, internal organs (such as the respiratory tract, gastrointestinal tract, and genitals), and areas of the body that are exposed to the external environment (such as the nostrils, eyes, lips, ears, and anus). They secrete mucus to maintain moisture and lubrication. Occasionally, certain inflammatory substances can irritate these membranes and cause them to produce excess mucus, which leads to congestion.

Recommendations include ascertaining the precipitating factors or causes of the congestion, avoiding mucus-producing foods such as dairy products, using drainage products to facilitate proper drainage of the congestion, the addition of lymphatic drainage therapies (a manual form of stimulating the drainage of the lymph system), increasing hydration and rest, and supplementation with enzymes and nutrients to support the immune system. Enzymes can also be used to improve digestion, particularly of mucus-producing foods like dairy foods, and reduce inflammation and the excess production of mucus.

ENZYME SUPPLEMENTATION SUGGESTIONS:

*Mucolase Formula three times daily (if the mucus is colored)

Purpose: To reduce excess mucus produced by the body; particularly helpful in treating sinus and chest congestion
Each serving should contain approximately:

Mucolase	30 mg

Supporting enzymes:

Amylase blend	7,000 DU	Cellulase blend	200 CU
Protease blend	20,000 HUT	Xylanase	250 XU
Glucoamylase	25 AGU	Pectinase with Phytase	175 endo-PG
Beta-glucanase	30 BGU	Hemicellulase	30 HCU
Lipase blend	250 FCCFIP	Invertase	5 INVU
Alpha-galactosidase	50 GALU		

*High Protease Formula three times daily (to support the immune system)

Purpose: To help support immune function and assist in removing viruses, fungal forms, toxins, bacteria, and heavy metals
Each capsule should contain approximately:

Protease blend	150,000 HUT	Serratiopeptidase	25,000 units
Mucolase	8 mg	Nattokinase blend	400 FU
Catalase	50 baker units		

High Potency Digestive Formula or **Dairy Digesting Formula** with meals (to ensure dairy breakdown)

Purpose: To radically enhance the digestion and assimilation of food while reducing the body's need to produce digestive enzymes; the higher potency formula will average about three times the potency of the average digestive formula; an average formula may be substituted if three times the regular dose is taken

Each serving should contain approximately:

Amylase blend	22,000 DU	Alpha-galactosidase	450 GALU
Protease blend	80,000 HUT	Phytase	50 PU
Lipase blend	3,000 FCCFIP	Pectinase	50 AJDU
Cellulase blend	2,000 CU	Xylanase	500 XU
Invertase	80 IAU	Hemicellulase	30 HCU
Lactase	900 LacU	Beta-glucanase	25 BGU
Maltase	200 DP	L. acidophilus	250 million CFU
Glucoamylase	50 AGU		

Purpose: To help break down the common allergens in dairy, which includes lactose and casein

Each serving should contain approximately:

Lactase	9,000 ALU	Amylase blend	7,500 DU
Protease blend	25,000 HUT	Glucoamylase	25 AG
Lipase blend	500 FCCFIP	Malstase	350 DP
Cellulase	300 CU		

High Amylase Formula three times daily (if the mucus is clear)

Purpose: To overcome symptoms of allergies and for the proper digestion of carbohydrates, especially grains, raw vegetables, and legumes

Each serving should contain approximately:

Amylase blend	22,000 DU	Cellulase blend	400 CU
Glucoamylase	30 AGU	Lactase	300 LacU
Alpha-galactosidase	1,000 GALU	Maltase	300 DP
Protease blend	15,000 HUT	Pectinase	20 endo-PG
Lipase blend	150 FCCFIP		

MULTIPLE SCLEROSIS

Multiple sclerosis (MS) is a chronic disease that affects the central nervous system. This progressive, degenerative disease involves the gradual loss of the myelin sheath that surrounds and protects the nerve fibers in the body. With the loss of the myelin, the nerve fibers become scarred, disrupting communication between the brain and other parts of the body. While the cause of MS is not known, some researchers believe that it is an autoimmune disorder.

Multiple sclerosis can cause a variety of symptoms including dizziness, sudden and transient sensory and motor disturbances, tingling sensation in parts of the body, visual problems, muscle weakness, nausea, depression, difficulties with coordination and speech, tremors, loss of bladder sensation, and loss of sexual function. The symptoms often come and go as "attacks," allowing many patients to lead full and rewarding lives. However, MS can cause impaired mobility and physical disability in more severe cases.

Primarily affecting adults, most cases of MS begin between twenty and forty years of age. Although there is no conclusive cause of MS, the following factors have been demonstrated to contribute to this disease: viral infection (e.g., measles), autoimmune reactions, a reduced capacity to detoxify free radicals, excessive lipid peroxidation, an excessive intake of saturated fatty acids and animal fats, and heavy metal toxicity.

Recommendations primarily include treating the symptoms of MS and supporting the overall health of the body through a healthy diet of natural foods, eliminating exposure to allergens as much as possible, and possibly treatment with certain drugs to limit the severity of attacks and the progression of the disease. Enzymes can be used to improve digestion and nutrient absorption, reduce inflammation and pain during attacks, strengthen the immune system, and balance the pH levels to support overall health.

ENZYME SUPPLEMENTATION SUGGESTIONS:

*High Potency Digestive Formula with every meal

Purpose: To radically enhance the digestion and assimilation of food while reducing the body's need to produce digestive enzymes; the higher potency formula will average about three times the potency of the average digestive formula; an average formula may be substituted if three times the regular dose is taken

Each serving should contain approximately:

Amylase blend	22,000 DU	Alpha-galactosidase	450 GALU
Protease blend	80,000 HUT	Phytase	50 PU
Lipase blend	3,000 FCCFIP	Pectinase	50 AJDU
Cellulase blend	2,000 CU	Xylanase	500 XU
Invertase	80 IAU	Hemicellulase	30 HCU
Lactase	900 LacU	Beta-glucanase	25 BGU
Maltase	200 DP	*L. acidophilus*	250 million CFU
Glucoamylase	50 AGU		

*High Lipase Formula three times daily with essential fatty acid supplements such as flax oil and fish oil.

Purpose: To improve fat digestion and metabolism, as well as the health of the cardiovascular system

Each capsule should contain approximately:

Lipase blend	5,000 FCCFIP	Protease blend	20,000 HUT
Amylase blend	10,000 DU	Lactase	300 LacU

*High Protease Formula three times daily

Purpose: To help support immune function and assist in removing viruses, fungal forms, toxins, bacteria, and heavy metals
Each capsule should contain approximately:

Protease blend	150,000 HUT	Serratiopeptidase	25,000 units
Mucolase	8 mg	Nattokinase blend	400 FU
Catalase	50 baker units		

pH Balancing Formula three times daily

Purpose: To help the body achieve an optimal pH
Each serving should contain approximately:

Amylase blend	25,000 DU	Lipase blend	175 FCCFIP
Cellulase blend	6,000 CU	Pectinase/Phytase	200 PU
Mineral blend	Potassium bicarbonate, sodium bicarbonate, magnesium citrate	Herbal blend	Hydrilla, marshmallow, papaya
Protease blend	1,000 HUT		

The formula should not exceed 8.0 on the pH scale and the capsule should be enteric coated.

Anti-inflammatory Formula anytime needed for inflammation or pain

Purpose: To address inflammation, speed recovery, and repair tissue; best if enteric coated
Each serving should contain approximately:

Protease blend	120,000 HUT	Amylase blend	7,000 DU
Papain	140,000 PU	Lipase blend	600 FCCFIP
Bromelain	1,200 GDU (11.25 million FCCPU)	Catalase	100 baker units

NAUSEA

Nausea is not an illness in itself; it is typically a symptom of another condition, which may not be related to the stomach at all. In fact, more often than not, nausea indicates a condition somewhere else in the body rather than in the stomach itself. Nausea can be caused by a variety of factors including reaction to certain foods, gallbladder imbalances, pregnancy, overeating, a reaction to certain medications, drugs, other therapies, or a heightened sensitivity to motion, such as occurs when riding in an automobile, boat, or airplane. Occasionally the stomach becomes upset as a result of these other conditions, creating the sensation of a need to vomit. Additional symptoms related to nausea may include excessive salivation, pallor, and sweating.

Enzymes can soothe the digestive system and maintain proper functioning.

ENZYME SUPPLEMENTATION SUGGESTIONS:

*High Potency Digestive Formula with every meal

Purpose: To radically enhance the digestion and assimilation of food while reducing the body's need to produce digestive enzymes; the higher potency formula will average about three times the potency of the average digestive formula; an average formula may be substituted if three times the regular dose is taken
    Each serving should contain approximately:

Amylase blend	22,000 DU	Alpha-galactosidase	450 GALU
Protease blend	80,000 HUT	Phytase	50 PU
Lipase blend	3,000 FCCFIP	Pectinase	50 AJDU
Cellulase blend	2,000 CU	Xylanase	500 XU
Invertase	80 IAU	Hemicellulase	30 HCU
Lactase	900 LacU	Beta-glucanase	25 BGU
Maltase	200 DP	L. acidophilus	250 million CFU
Glucoamylase	50 AGU		

*Soothing Digestive Formula after meals or any time it is needed

Purpose: To help alleviate conditions associated with gastrointestinal distress
    Each serving should contain approximately:

Amylase blend	2,000 DU	Gotu kola	50 mg
Lipase blend	175 FCCFIP	Papaya leaf	100 mg
Cellulase blend	400 CU	Prickly ash bark	50 mg
Marshmallow root	100 mg		

Additional helpful ingredients:

DGL (deglycyrrhizinated licorice)	

This formula should *not* contain protease. Other herbs may also be present.

NERVOUSNESS

See STRESS or ANXIETY.

OSTEOPOROSIS

Osteoporosis is a general loss of bone density. The major cause of osteoporosis is the gradual loss of protein matrix tissue from the bone. This loss results in weakened bones, which can cause pain in the back and hips, loss of height, increased risk of fractures, and spinal curvature. The underlying mechanism in all cases of osteoporosis is an imbalance between bone resorption and bone formation. Bone undergoes a constant process of formation (using nutrients and particularly minerals absorbed by the body) and resorption (the process by which the body breaks bone down to absorb calcium into the blood). Resorption is regulated based on the amount of calcium in the body. In osteoporosis, either bone resorption is excessive, or bone formation is diminished. While consuming enough calcium is important, there are other factors involved in osteoporosis that affect the process of absorbing calcium and using it to generate bone mass.

Osteoporosis afflicts more women than men, particularly postmenopausal women, since their ovaries are no longer producing estrogen, which helps to maintain bone mass. Osteoporosis is also more common in smokers and drinkers and is associated with chronic obstructive lung disorders, such as emphysema and bronchitis. Additional causative factors include lack of exercise, a calcium-phosphorus imbalance, lactose intolerance, and a diminished ability to absorb calcium through the intestines. Approximately 15 to 20 million Americans suffer from this disorder.

While treatments are becoming available, prevention is still the most important way to reduce the effects of osteoporosis. Enzyme therapy can be used to improve digestion and absorption of nutrients, particularly calcium; stimulate the immune system; balance the pH levels; improve hormone regulation (particularly during menopause); and reduce inflammation when inflammation and pain occur.

ENZYME SUPPLEMENTATION SUGGESTIONS:

*High Potency Digestive Formula or Dairy Digesting Formula (if lactose intolerant)

Purpose: To radically enhance the digestion and assimilation of food while reducing the body's need to produce digestive enzymes; the higher potency formula will average about three times the potency of the average digestive formula; an average formula may be substituted if three times the regular dose is taken

Each serving should contain approximately:

Amylase blend	22,000 DU	Alpha-galactosidase	450 GALU
Protease blend	80,000 HUT	Phytase	50 PU
Lipase blend	3,000 FCCFIP	Pectinase	50 AJDU
Cellulase blend	2,000 CU	Xylanase	500 XU
Invertase	80 IAU	Hemicellulase	30 HCU
Lactase	900 LacU	Beta-glucanase	25 BGU
Maltase	200 DP	L. acidophilus	250 million CFU
Glucoamylase	50 AGU		

Purpose: To help break down the common allergens in dairy, which includes lactose and casein

Each serving should contain approximately:

Lactase	9,000 ALU	Amylase blend	7,500 DU
Protease blend	25,000 HUT	Glucoamylase	25 AG
Lipase blend	500 FCCFIP	Malstase	350 DP
Cellulase	300 CU		

*pH Balancing Formula three times daily

Purpose: To help the body achieve an optimal pH

Each serving should contain approximately:

Amylase blend	25,000 DU	Lipase blend	175 FCCFIP
Cellulase blend	6,000 CU	Pectinase/Phytase	200 PU
Mineral blend	Potassium bicarbonate, sodium bicarbonate, magnesium citrate	Herbal blend	Hydrilla, marshmallow, papaya
Protease blend	1,000 HUT		

The formula should not exceed 8.0 on the pH scale and the capsule should be enteric coated.

High Lipase Formula three times daily

Purpose: To improve fat digestion and metabolism, and support the endocrine system in production of hormones

Each capsule should contain approximately:

Lipase blend	5,000 FCCFIP	Protease blend	20,000 HUT
Amylase blend	10,000 DU	Lactase	300 LacU

High Protease Formula three times per day

Purpose: To help support immune function and assist in removing viruses, fungal forms, toxins, bacteria, and heavy metals
  Each capsule should contain approximately:

Protease blend	150,000 HUT	Serratiopeptidase	25,000 units
Mucolase	8 mg	Nattokinase blend	400 FU
Catalase	50 baker units		

Anti-inflammatory Formula anytime inflammation or pain occurs

Purpose: To address inflammation, speed recovery, and repair tissue; best if enteric coated
  Each serving should contain approximately:

Protease blend	120,000 HUT	Amylase blend	7,000 DU
Papain	140,000 PU	Lipase blend	600 FCCFIP
Bromelain	1,200 GDU (11.25 million FCCPU)	Catalase	100 baker units

OXIDATIVE STRESS

Oxidative stress is a medical term for damage to animal or plant cells (and thereby the organs and tissues composed of those cells) caused by reactive oxygen ions. It is defined as an imbalance between pro-oxidants and antioxidants, with the former prevailing. Oxidative stress is thought to contribute to the aging process.

Compounds that prevent free-radical damage are known as antioxidants. The body produces antioxidant enzymes, including catalase, glutathione peroxidase, and super oxide dismutase (SOD). These enzymes prevent damage caused by certain types of free radicals.

Symptoms of free radical damage (necessitating dietary antioxidant therapies) can include but are not limited to headaches, frequent or chronic infections, palpitations, neck spasms, back pain, inability to relax, chronic allergies, diarrhea, nausea, heavy metal toxicity, and chronic yeast infections or candidiasis.

Laboratory studies are demonstrating that ingesting higher levels of antioxidants can increase life expectancy. Research is indicating that increasing levels of these compounds, which include vitamins C and E, betacarotene, selenium, coenzyme Q10, flavonoids, and sulfur-containing amino acids (cystein and methionine), can reduce the risk of cancer, heart disease, arthritis, macular degeneration, and other age-related degenerative conditions.

Enzymes can support the digestion and absorption of nutrients; fight the effects of free radicals in the body (particularly if the enzymes are proteases) improve pH balance; and reduce inflammation, which can be a side effect of free radical damage.

ENZYME SUPPLEMENTATION SUGGESTIONS:

*High Potency Digestive Formula with every meal

Purpose: To radically enhance the digestion and assimilation of food while reducing the body's need to produce digestive enzymes; the higher potency formula will average about three times the potency of the average digestive formula; an average formula may be substituted if three times the regular dose is taken

Each serving should contain approximately:

Amylase blend	22,000 DU	Alpha-galactosidase	450 GALU
Protease blend	80,000 HUT	Phytase	50 PU
Lipase blend	3,000 FCCFIP	Pectinase	50 AJDU
Cellulase blend	2,000 CU	Xylanase	500 XU
Invertase	80 IAU	Hemicellulase	30 HCU
Lactase	900 LacU	Beta-glucanase	25 BGU
Maltase	200 DP	L. acidophilus	250 million CFU
Glucoamylase	50 AGU		

*Antioxidant Supplement two times daily on an empty stomach

Purpose: To reduce oxidative stress

Each serving should contain approximately:

SOD (superoxide dismutase)	75 mg	Catalase	250 baker units
Protease blend	50,000 HUT	Alpha Lopoic acid	100 mg
Glutathione	60 mg		

High Protease Formula three times daily

Purpose: To help support immune function and assist in removing viruses, fungal forms, toxins, bacteria, and heavy metals

Each capsule should contain approximately:

Protease blend	150,000 HUT	Serratiopeptidase	25,000 units
Mucolase	8 mg	Nattokinase blend	400 FU
Catalase	50 baker units		

pH Balancing Formula three times daily

Purpose: To help the body achieve an optimal pH
    Each serving should contain approximately:

Amylase blend	25,000 DU	Lipase blend	175 FCCFIP
Cellulase blend	6,000 CU	Pectinase/Phytase	200 PU
Mineral blend	Potassium bicarbonate, sodium bicarbonate, magnesium citrate	Herbal blend	Hydrilla, marshmallow, papaya
Protease blend	1,000 HUT		

The formula should not exceed 8.0 on the pH scale and the capsule should be enteric coated.

PARASITES

Any organism that spends a significant portion of its life in or on the living tissue of a host organism and that causes harm to the host without immediately killing it is a parasite. Parasites typically show highly specialized adaptations that allow them to exploit host resources. Some parasites cause minor symptoms, while others can cause extensive disease.

There are two kinds of parasites: endoparasites (those that live within their hosts), which include fungi (such as RINGWORM) and protozoa (such as *Giardia lamblia*); and ectoparasites (those that live on but not within their hosts), which include ticks, fleas, and lice.

Viruses and disease-causing fungi and bacteria are all considered parasites, and all have an outer coating of protein. After they have been targeted by the immune system as a foreign agent, the cells of the immune system begin to remove them (see chapter 2).

Enzymes can support the immune system's efforts to remove parasitic cells from the body. Proteases in the bloodstream are used by the immune system to break down the protein cell structure to allow the immune cells to destroy the parasites. In addition, enzymes can promote overall health by balancing pH levels. A probiotic formula can improve an imbalance of bacteria in the intestines.

ENZYME SUPPLEMENTATION SUGGESTIONS:

*High Potency Digestive Formula with every meal

Purpose: To radically enhance the digestion and assimilation of food while reducing the body's need to produce digestive enzymes; the higher potency formula will average about three times the potency of the average digestive formula; an average formula may be substituted if three times the regular dose is taken

Each serving should contain approximately:

Amylase blend	22,000 DU	Alpha-galactosidase	450 GALU
Protease blend	80,000 HUT	Phytase	50 PU
Lipase blend	3,000 FCCFIP	Pectinase	50 AJDU
Cellulase blend	2,000 CU	Xylanase	500 XU
Invertase	80 IAU	Hemicellulase	30 HCU
Lactase	900 LacU	Beta-glucanase	25 BGU
Maltase	200 DP	L. acidophilus	250 million CFU
Glucoamylase	50 AGU		

*High Protease Formula three to four times daily on an empty stomach

Purpose: To help support immune function and assist in removing viruses, fungal forms, toxins, bacteria, and heavy metals
Each capsule should contain approximately:

Protease blend	150,000 HUT	Serratiopeptidase	25,000 units
Mucolase	8 mg	Nattokinase blend	400 FU
Catalase	50 baker units		

*Probiotic Formula daily before bed

Purpose: To assist the body in balancing microflora
Each serving should contain approximately 5 billion probiotic live cells (guaranteed potency), comprised of:

Bacillus Subtillis	No less than 3 billion CFU guaranteed potency	A blend of L. acidophilus, L. casei, L. bulgaris, L. plantarum, L. rhamnosus, L. salivarius	No less than 1 billion CFU guaranteed potency
L. paracassei F-19	No less than 1 billion CFU guaranteed potency		

pH Balancing Formula three times daily

Purpose: To help the body achieve an optimal pH
Each serving should contain approximately:

Amylase blend	25,000 DU	Lipase blend	175 FCCFIP
Cellulase blend	6,000 CU	Pectinase/Phytase	200 PU
Mineral blend	Potassium bicarbonate, sodium bicarbonate, magnesium citrate	Herbal blend	Hydrilla, marshmallow, papaya
Protease blend	1,000 HUT		

The formula should not exceed 8.0 on the pH scale and the capsule should be enteric coated.

PEPTIC ULCER

A peptic ulcer is a sore on the mucous membrane of the gastrointestinal tract occurring in the esophagus, stomach, or duodenum. Ulcers in the colon are usually referred to as ulcerative colitis. (See INFLAMMATORY BOWEL DISEASE.) Ulcers are characterized by damage to and loss of tissue in the affected area. They are also vulnerable to secondary infection by bacteria, fungi, or viruses. Ulcers can take a long time to heal and result in a generalized weakness of the patient and the immune system.

Symptoms of peptic ulcers can include abdominal tenderness and abdominal distress within an hour after meals or during the night. This distress is often relieved by ingesting food, taking antacids, or vomiting. Other symptoms may include vomiting blood, weight loss, or foul-smelling feces. Factors that can cause peptic ulcers include stress, smoking, poor diet, and food allergies.

Enzymes can be used to improve digestion, soothe the digestive tract, and balance the pH levels in the body to manage possible overproduction or underproduction of stomach acids. (See also INDIGESTION or GASTROESOPHAGEAL REFLUX.)

ENZYME SUPPLEMENTATION SUGGESTIONS:

*High Amylase Formula with every meal

Purpose: For the proper digestion of carbohydrates, especially grains, raw vegetables, and legumes

Each serving should contain approximately:

Amylase blend	22,000 DU	Cellulase blend	400 CU
Glucoamylase	30 AGU	Lactase	300 LacU
Alpha-galactosidase	1,000 GALU	Maltase	300 DP
Protease blend	15,000 HUT	Pectinase	20 endo-PG
Lipase blend	150 FCCFIP		

*Soothing Digestive Formula after every meal or taken as needed

Purpose: To help alleviate conditions associated with gastrointestinal distress
Each serving should contain approximately:

Amylase blend	2,000 DU	Gotu kola	50 mg
Lipase blend	175 FCCFIP	Papaya leaf	100 mg
Cellulase blend	400 CU	Prickly ash bark	50 mg
Marshmallow root	100 mg		

Additional helpful ingredients:

DGL (deglycyrrhizinated licorice)	

This formula should *not* contain protease. Other herbs may also be present.

*pH Balancing Formula three times daily

Purpose: To help the body achieve an optimal pH
Each serving should contain approximately:

Amylase blend	25,000 DU	Lipase blend	175 FCCFIP
Cellulase blend	6,000 CU	Pectinase/Phytase	200 PU
Mineral blend	Potassium bicarbonate, sodium bicarbonate, magnesium citrate	Herbal blend	Hydrilla, marshmallow, papaya
Protease blend	1,000 HUT		

The formula should not exceed 8.0 on the pH scale and the capsule should be enteric coated.

PERIODONTAL DISORDERS

Anyone who has had a periodontal disorder will tell you how important it is to take care of your teeth and gums. Periodontal disorders can include bleeding gums, gingivitis, and pyorrhea. These conditions can worsen and progress over time, resulting in infection, tooth loss, and major interventions, including extractions and surgeries.

An early stage of periodontal disease, gingivitis is a condition that involves an inflammation of the gums. Deposits of food particles, mucus, and bacteria often cause an accumulation of plaque. Gingivitis is the accumulation of plaque around the teeth that causes the gum tissue to become swollen, red, and infected. The gums often bleed. Aside from poor dental maintenance and care, a poor diet, poorly fitted fillings that irritate the gums, and frequent breathing through the mouth can also aggravate or cause gingivitis.

If gingivitis goes untreated, it can develop into periodontitis. This ailment is also often related to a deficiency of calcium, folic acid, niacin, bioflavonoid, or vitamin C. Additional causes of periodontitis may include poor diet, chronic illness, blood disease, smoking, drugs, and excessive alcohol consumption.

In general, the symptoms of periodontal disorders or disease can include one or more of the following: infection, abscesses, pain and inflammation in the gums, halitosis (bad breath), and in severe cases, infection of the bone resulting in bone destruction. (See also CANKER SORES.)

Recommendations include regular dental care; regular brushing and flossing; a healthy, well-balanced diet; elimination of toxic agents (smoking, alcohol, excess sugar); and nutritional support. Enzymes can improve digestion and nutrient absorption, support the immune system, and maintain balanced pH levels.

ENZYME SUPPLEMENTATION SUGGESTIONS:

*High Potency Digestive Formula with every meal

Purpose: To radically enhance the digestion and assimilation of food while reducing the body's need to produce digestive enzymes; the higher potency formula will average about three times the potency of the average digestive formula; an average formula may be substituted if three times the regular dose is taken
Each serving should contain approximately:

Amylase blend	22,000 DU	Alpha-galactosidase	450 GALU
Protease blend	80,000 HUT	Phytase	50 PU
Lipase blend	3,000 FCCFIP	Pectinase	50 AJDU
Cellulase blend	2,000 CU	Xylanase	500 XU
Invertase	80 IAU	Hemicellulase	30 HCU
Lactase	900 LacU	Beta-glucanase	25 BGU
Maltase	200 DP	L. acidophilus	250 million CFU
Glucoamylase	50 AGU		

*Serratiopeptidase Formula two times daily

Purpose: To break down protein and reduce inflammation. Also supports cardiovascular health and enhances other proteases.

Each serving should contain approximately:

Serratiopeptidase	80,000 SU
Protease blend	70,000 HUT
Mineral blend	50 mg

Supporting enzymes:

Bromelain	Papain

*pH Balancing Formula three times daily

Purpose: To help the body achieve an optimal pH

Each serving should contain approximately:

Amylase blend	25,000 DU	Lipase blend	175 FCCFIP
Cellulase blend	6,000 CU	Pectinase/Phytase	200 PU
Mineral blend	Potassium bicarbonate, sodium bicarbonate, magnesium citrate	Herbal blend	Hydrilla, marshmallow, papaya
Protease blend	1,000 HUT		

The formula should not exceed 8.0 on the pH scale and the capsule should be enteric coated.

High Protease Formula three times daily

Purpose: To help support immune function and assist in removing viruses, fungal forms, toxins, bacteria, and heavy metals

Each capsule should contain approximately:

Protease blend	150,000 HUT	Serratiopeptidase	25,000 units
Mucolase	8 mg	Nattokinase blend	400 FU
Catalase	50 baker units		

High Amylase Formula may be added when consuming any high-carbohydrate or high-sugar foods

Purpose: To overcome symptoms of allergies and for the proper digestion of carbohydrates, especially grains, raw vegetables, and legumes

Each serving should contain approximately:

Amylase blend	22,000 DU	Cellulase blend	400 CU
Glucoamylase	30 AGU	Lactase	300 LacU
Alpha-galactosidase	1,000 GALU	Maltase	300 DP
Protease blend	15,000 HUT	Pectinase	20 endo-PG
Lipase blend	150 FCCFIP		

PITUITARY IMBALANCES

The pituitary gland is a pea-size structure that hangs from the base of the brain. This gland helps control aspects of physical growth, blood pressure (see HYPERTENSION), pregnancy (including breast milk production), thyroid and adrenal gland function (see HYPOTHYROIDISM or ADRENAL INSUFFICIENCY), and overall metabolism.

Any abnormality of this gland usually means that it produces either too much or too little of one or more hormones and is causing changes elsewhere in the body. The hormones that may be affected include ACHT, which stimulates hormone production by the adrenal glands; an antidiuretic hormone, which acts on the kidneys to decrease water loss in the urine and thus reduces urine volume; TSH, which is the hormone that stimulates the thyroid; the growth hormone, prolactin, which stimulates female breast development; melanocyte, which helps control the function of male and female sex organs; and oxytocin, which stimulates contraction of the uterus during childbirth and milk release from the breasts.

To support the health of the pituitary gland, enzymes can be used to improve digestion and nutrient absorption, support the proper functioning of the immune system, and improve hormonal balance.

ENZYME SUPPLEMENTATION SUGGESTIONS:

*High Potency Digestive Formula with every meal

Purpose: To radically enhance the digestion and assimilation of food while reducing the body's need to produce digestive enzymes; the higher potency formula will average about three times the potency of the average digestive formula; an average formula may be substituted if three times the regular dose is taken

Each serving should contain approximately:

Amylase blend	22,000 DU	Alpha-galactosidase	450 GALU
Protease blend	80,000 HUT	Phytase	50 PU
Lipase blend	3,000 FCCFIP	Pectinase	50 AJDU
Cellulase blend	2,000 CU	Xylanase	500 XU
Invertase	80 IAU	Hemicellulase	30 HCU
Lactase	900 LacU	Beta-glucanase	25 BGU
Maltase	200 DP	L. acidophilus	250 million CFU
Glucoamylase	50 AGU		

*High Lipase Formula three times daily

Purpose: To improve fat digestion and metabolism, and support the endocrine system in the production of hormones
Each capsule should contain approximately:

Lipase blend	5,000 FCCFIP	Protease blend	20,000 HUT
Amylase blend	10,000 DU	Lactase	300 LacU

High Protease Formula three to four times daily

Purpose: To help support immune function and assist in removing viruses, fungal forms, toxins, bacteria, and heavy metals
Each capsule should contain approximately:

Protease blend	150,000 HUT	Serratiopeptidase	25,000 units
Mucolase	8 mg	Nattokinase blend	400 FU
Catalase	50 baker units		

PREMENSTRUAL SYNDROME

Premenstrual syndrome (PMS) is the combination of various physical and emotional symptoms that occur in women during the week or two before menstruation begins. This syndrome affects more than 75 percent of women of reproductive age at some point during their lifetime, although it occurs most often in women between their late twenties and early forties. In a smaller percentage of women, the symptoms are severe and interfere with their regular functioning. This condition is called premenstrual dysphoric disorder and is characterized by severe depression, irritability, and tension.

Hormonal changes that occur throughout the menstrual cycle clearly influence PMS, but there is no established, concrete cause for the symptoms. PMS may cause mood swings, irritability, tension, depression, anxiety, and fatigue. Physical symptoms may include breast tenderness, fluid retention, headaches, backaches, cramping, bloating, and lower abdominal pain. Fluid retention, directly linked to fluctuations in estrogen levels, has been associated with other symptoms, and if fluid retention can be reduced, other symptoms seem to lessen.

Recommendations include eating a healthy, well-balanced diet; getting regular exercise (which has been shown to reduce the symptoms of PMS by maintaining more balanced hormone levels and reducing fluid retention); or reducing/managing stress; and getting adequate rest and sleep. Enzymes can maintain digestion and nutrient absorption and balance hormone levels in the body.

ENZYME SUPPLEMENTATION SUGGESTIONS:

*High Potency Digestive Formula with every meal

Purpose: To radically enhance the digestion and assimilation of food while reducing the body's need to produce digestive enzymes; the higher potency formula will average about three times the potency of the average digestive formula; an average formula may be substituted if three times the regular dose is taken

Each serving should contain approximately:

Amylase blend	22,000 DU	Alpha-galactosidase	450 GALU
Protease blend	80,000 HUT	Phytase	50 PU
Lipase blend	3,000 FCCFIP	Pectinase	50 AJDU
Cellulase blend	2,000 CU	Xylanase	500 XU
Invertase	80 IAU	Hemicellulase	30 HCU
Lactase	900 LacU	Beta-glucanase	25 BGU
Maltase	200 DP	L. acidophilus	250 million CFU
Glucoamylase	50 AGU		

*High Lipase Formula three times daily

Purpose: To improve fat digestion and metabolism, and support the endocrine system in the production of hormones

Each capsule should contain approximately:

Lipase blend	5,000 FCCFIP	Protease blend	20,000 HUT
Amylase blend	10,000 DU	Lactase	300 LacU

High Protease Formula three times daily

Purpose: To help support immune function and assist in removing viruses, fungal forms, toxins, bacteria, and heavy metals
    Each capsule should contain approximately:

Protease blend	150,000 HUT	Serratiopeptidase	25,000 units
Mucolase	8 mg	Nattokinase blend	400 FU
Catalase	50 baker units		

PROSTATE DISORDERS

The prostate is the male sex gland that is positioned beneath the bladder. This doughnut-shaped gland encircles the urethra where it connects to the bladder. Both urine and semen pass through the prostate. During ejaculation, the muscles in the prostate squeeze seminal fluids into the urethral tract. Disorders of the prostate rarely occur before the age of thirty.

Prostate problems include benign prostatic hypertrophy (BPH), which results in an enlarged prostate that can narrow the urethra; prostatitis, acute or chronic inflammation of the prostate gland; and cancer.

Benign prostatic hypertrophy occurs in all men as they age, although it is not known why the prostate enlarges over time. Symptoms of prostate enlargement can include frequent urination, especially during the night; pelvic pain; burning; impotence; and difficulty starting and stopping urination. Problems urinating can lead to urine remaining and becoming stagnant in the bladder, causing infection of the bladder and the kidneys. See also BLADDER INFECTION and KIDNEY STRESS.

Symptoms of prostatitis include fever, frequent urination accompanied by a burning sensation, blood or pus in the urine, urinary tract infection, and pain between the scrotum and the rectum. As prostatitis becomes more severe, urination can become difficult.

Prostate cancer rarely occurs in men under sixty years of age. Symptoms are vague and can include difficulty in starting urination, blood in the urine, a burning sensation during urination, and increasing frequency of urination at night. The symptoms can be mistaken for the problems associated with an enlarged prostate.

Recommendations for maintaining prostate, bladder, and kidney health include thorough prostate examinations every year for men over forty years of age, dietary changes (including avoiding foods with a high fat content), regular exercise, and increased water intake. Enzymes can improve digestion and nutrient absorption, improve circulation, improve digestion of fats, and balance pH levels.

ENZYME SUPPLEMENTATION SUGGESTIONS:

*High Potency Digestive Formula

Purpose: To radically enhance the digestion and assimilation of food while reducing the body's need to produce digestive enzymes; the higher potency formula will average about three times the potency of the average digestive formula; an average formula may be substituted if three times the regular dose is taken
    Each serving should contain approximately:

Amylase blend	22,000 DU	Alpha-galactosidase	450 GALU
Protease blend	80,000 HUT	Phytase	50 PU
Lipase blend	3,000 FCCFIP	Pectinase	50 AJDU
Cellulase blend	2,000 CU	Xylanase	500 XU
Invertase	80 IAU	Hemicellulase	30 HCU
Lactase	900 LacU	Beta-glucanase	25 BGU
Maltase	200 DP	L. acidophilus	250 million CFU
Glucoamylase	50 AGU		

*Nattokinase Formula three times daily

Purpose: To decrease blood pressure by breaking down fibrin, reduce inflammation
    Each serving should contain approximately:
    Necessary ingredient:

Nattokinase NSK-SD	1,000 FU

Helpful ingredients:

Amylase blend	9,000 DU	Glucoamylase	25 AGU
Protease blend	20,000 HUT	Lipase blend	1,000 FCCFIP
Minerals	85 mg	Cellulase blend	400 CU

High Lipase Formula three times daily

Purpose: To improve fat digestion and metabolism, and support the endocrine system in the production of hormones
    Each capsule should contain approximately:

Lipase blend	5,000 FCCFIP	Protease blend	20,000 HUT
Amylase blend	10,000 DU	Lactase	300 LacU

Serratiopeptidase Formula may be added to the nattokinase formula for better results

Purpose: To break down protein and reduce inflammation. Also supports cardiovascular health and enhances other proteases.

Each serving should contain approximately:

Serratiopeptidase	80,000 SU
Protease blend	70,000 HUT
Mineral blend	50 mg

Supporting enzymes:

Bromelain	Papain

PSORIASIS

Psoriasis is a chronic skin disease marked by red, scaly patches. With psoriasis, skin cells form too quickly and are replaced by new cells before they can mature. No one knows why this skin cell turnover takes place at such a rapid rate. For some reason, possibly due to an autoimmune reaction, the skin loses its ability to regulate the production of skin cells.

Factors such as injury to the skin, prescription drugs, stress, cold weather, bacterial infections, surgery, or sunburn may trigger psoriasis. The immune system may play a key role in the defense against the development of psoriasis.

Recommendations include digestive enzyme therapy to improve the digestion of food, maintain normal pH levels, and detoxify the body. Systemic enzyme therapy can support the immune system and act as a natural anti-inflammatory. Finally, proteolytic enzymes may help to improve circulation, speed tissue repair, and enhance wellness.

ENZYME SUPPLEMENTATION SUGGESTIONS:

*High Potency Digestive Formula with every meal

Purpose: To radically enhance the digestion and assimilation of food while reducing the body's need to produce digestive enzymes; the higher potency formula will average about three times the potency of the average digestive formula; an average formula may be substituted if three times the regular dose is taken

Each serving should contain approximately:

Amylase blend	22,000 DU	Alpha-galactosidase	450 GALU
Protease blend	80,000 HUT	Phytase	50 PU
Lipase blend	3,000 FCCFIP	Pectinase	50 AJDU
Cellulase blend	2,000 CU	Xylanase	500 XU
Invertase	80 IAU	Hemicellulase	30 HCU
Lactase	900 LacU	Beta-glucanase	25 BGU
Maltase	200 DP	L. acidophilus	250 million CFU
Glucoamylase	50 AGU		

*High Protease Formula three to four times daily

Purpose: To help support immune function and assist in removing viruses, fungal forms, toxins, bacteria, and heavy metals

Each capsule should contain approximately:

Protease blend	150,000 HUT	Serratiopeptidase	25,000 units
Mucolase	8 mg	Nattokinase blend	400 FU
Catalase	50 baker units		

Serratiopeptidase Formula may be added for anti-inflammatory support

Purpose: To break down protein and reduce inflammation. Also supports cardiovascular health and enhances other proteases.

Each serving should contain approximately:

Serratiopeptidase	80,000 SU
Protease blend	70,000 HUT
Mineral blend	50 mg

Supporting enzymes:

Bromelain	Papain

High Lipase Formula whenever flax oil or fish oil supplements are taken

Purpose: To improve fat digestion and metabolism, as well as the health of the cardio-vascular system

Each capsule should contain approximately:

Lipase blend	5,000 FCCFIP	Protease blend	20,000 HUT
Amylase blend	10,000 DU	Lactase	300 LacU

RESPIRATORY AILMENTS

See ALLERGIES, ASTHMA, and BRONCHITIS.

RHEUMATISM

See ARTHRITIS.

RINGWORM

Ringworm (*tinea*) is a fungal skin infection that can affect various parts of the body. The different types of ringworm are classified by the areas of the body they infect. Ringworm on general areas of the body (arms, legs, trunk) is called *tinea corporis*; ringworm on the scalp is called *tinea capitis*; ringworm in the groin area is called *tinea cruris* (also called jock itch); and ringworm on the feet is called *tinea pedis* (or athlete's foot).

Ringworm typically appears as itchy, red, raised, scaly patches of skin that may blister and ooze. The patches often have sharply defined edges that are redder than in the center, which creates the appearance of a ring. The skin may also appear unusually dark or light. When the scalp or beard is infected, ringworm causes round bald patches. If the nails are infected, they can become discolored, thick, and even crumble. Athlete's foot usually occurs between the toes. It is particularly prevalent and highly contagious in damp, warm places, such as locker rooms, swimming pools, showers, and gyms.

Recommendations for treating ringworm include eating a well-balanced diet and reducing intake of foods that are high in sugar, which can support the overgrowth of fungus in the body. Enzyme therapy is used to support the immune and digestive systems and reduce overgrowth of fungus.

ENZYME SUPPLEMENTATION SUGGESTIONS:

*High Potency Digestive Formula with every meal

Purpose: To radically enhance the digestion and assimilation of food while reducing the body's need to produce digestive enzymes; the higher potency formula will average about three times the potency of the average digestive formula; an average formula may be substituted if three times the regular dose is taken
     Each serving should contain approximately:

Amylase blend	22,000 DU	Alpha-galactosidase	450 GALU
Protease blend	80,000 HUT	Phytase	50 PU
Lipase blend	3,000 FCCFIP	Pectinase	50 AJDU
Cellulase blend	2,000 CU	Xylanase	500 XU
Invertase	80 IAU	Hemicellulase	30 HCU
Lactase	900 LacU	Beta-glucanase	25 BGU
Maltase	200 DP	L. acidophilus	250 million CFU
Glucoamylase	50 AGU		

*High Cellulase Formula three times daily between meals for one week

Purpose: To manage yeast overgrowth
     Each capsule should contain approximately:

Cellulase blend	30,000 CU
Protease blend	100,000 HUT

Contraindications: High amounts of cellulase should not be taken with certain timed-release medications that contain cellulose.

*High Protease Formula three times daily

Purpose: To help support immune function and assist in removing viruses, fungal forms, toxins, bacteria, and heavy metals
     Each capsule should contain approximately:

Protease blend	150,000 HUT	Serratiopeptidase	25,000 units
Mucolase	8 mg	Nattokinase blend	400 FU
Catalase	50 baker units		

*Probiotic Formula daily before bed

Purpose: To assist the body in balancing microflora

Each serving should contain approximately 5 billion probiotic live cells (guaranteed potency), comprised of:

Bacillus Subtillis	No less than 3 billion CFU guaranteed potency	A blend of *L. acidophilus, L. casei, L. bulgaris, L. plantarum, L. rhamnosus, L. salivarius*	No less than 1 billion CFU guaranteed potency
L. paracassei F-19	No less than 1 billion CFU guaranteed potency		

SHINGLES

See HERPES ZOSTER.

SINUSITIS

The sinuses are mucous membrane–lined air-filled cavities located in the facial region. These include the frontal sinuses, the maxillary sinuses, two sinus cavities located between the nasal cavity and eye sockets, and the collection of air spaces in the large, winged bone behind the nose that forms the central part of the base of the skull.

Sinusitis is an inflammation of the nasal sinuses that usually accompanies upper respiratory infections. This ailment is most frequently caused by bacterial infections, although it may be caused by viral infections as well. Smoking, irritating smells or fumes, nasal injuries, and growths in the nose may cause chronic sinusitis. Sinusitis can also be caused by allergic reactions, particularly to dairy products and airborne allergens. (See ALLERGIES.)

Symptoms can include but are not limited to nasal congestion, fever, facial pain, headache, earache, toothache, general malaise, cranial pressure, clear or green/yellow mucus discharge, and a loss of the sense of smell.

Recommendations include ascertaining the underlying cause of the sinusitis, ingesting hot liquids to relieve congestion and promote mucus flow, using various drainage techniques, and avoiding mucus-producing foods, such as dairy products. Enzymes can be used to support digestion and nutrient absorption, reduce excess mucus, and combat the symptoms of allergies.

ENZYME SUPPLEMENTATION SUGGESTIONS:

*Mucolase Formula three times daily

Purpose: To reduce excess mucus produced by the body; particularly helpful in treating sinus and chest congestion

Each serving should contain approximately:

Mucolase	30 mg

Supporting enzymes:

Amylase blend	7,000 DU	Cellulase blend	200 CU
Protease blend	20,000 HUT	Xylanase	250 XU
Glucoamylase	25 AGU	Pectinase with Phytase	175 endo-PG
Beta-glucanase	30 BGU	Hemicellulase	30 HCU
Lipase blend	250 FCCFIP	Invertase	5 INVU
Alpha-galactosidase	50 GALU		

High Potency Digestive Formula with every meal

Purpose: To radically enhance the digestion and assimilation of food while reducing the body's need to produce digestive enzymes; the higher potency formula will average about three times the potency of the average digestive formula; an average formula may be substituted if three times the regular dose is taken

Each serving should contain approximately:

Amylase blend	22,000 DU	Alpha-galactosidase	450 GALU
Protease blend	80,000 HUT	Phytase	50 PU
Lipase blend	3,000 FCCFIP	Pectinase	50 AJDU
Cellulase blend	2,000 CU	Xylanase	500 XU
Invertase	80 IAU	Hemicellulase	30 HCU
Lactase	900 LacU	Beta-glucanase	25 BGU
Maltase	200 DP	L. acidophilus	250 million CFU
Glucoamylase	50 AGU		

High Amylase Formula may be added for allergy assistance

Purpose: To overcome symptoms of allergies and for the proper digestion of carbohydrates, especially grains, raw vegetables, and legumes

Each serving should contain approximately:

Amylase blend	22,000 DU	Cellulase blend	400 CU
Glucoamylase	30 AGU	Lactase	300 LacU
Alpha-galactosidase	1,000 GALU	Maltase	300 DP
Protease blend	15,000 HUT	Pectinase	20 endo-PG
Lipase blend	150 FCCFIP		

SKIN PROBLEMS

See ACNE, AGE SPOTS, DANDRUFF, DERMATITIS, HERPES VIRUS, HERPES ZOSTER, PSORIASIS, RINGWORM, or SKIN ULCERS.

SKIN ULCERS

Skin ulcers are areas of damaged skin and tissue that result in the loss of part or all of the upper skin tissue (not usually progressing below the dermis, or the deepest layer of the skin). Decubitus ulcers, also called bedsores, pressure sores, or pressure ulcers, develop when sustained pressure, usually from a bed or wheelchair, cuts off blood circulation to a particular area. Without adequate blood flow, the affected tissue dies. Bedsores are most commonly found on the hips, shoulder blades, buttocks, sacrum, and heels of comatose patients, the bedridden, and paraplegic patients. The best way to prevent bedsores is to turn or move patients regularly and ensure that their skin is clean.

Ulcers can also occur as a result of poor circulation (particularly with diabetes), infections of the skin, and sexually transmitted diseases.

Supporting the digestive and immune systems, controlling inflammation, and improving circulation to the affected areas is essential. Enzyme therapies can assist with all of these goals.

ENZYME SUPPLEMENTATION SUGGESTIONS:

*High Potency Digestive Formula with every meal

Purpose: To radically enhance the digestion and assimilation of food while reducing the body's need to produce digestive enzymes; the higher potency formula will average about three times the potency of the average digestive formula; an average formula may be substituted if three times the regular dose is taken

Each serving should contain approximately:

Amylase blend	22,000 DU	Alpha-galactosidase	450 GALU
Protease blend	80,000 HUT	Phytase	50 PU
Lipase blend	3,000 FCCFIP	Pectinase	50 AJDU
Cellulase blend	2,000 CU	Xylanase	500 XU
Invertase	80 IAU	Hemicellulase	30 HCU
Lactase	900 LacU	Beta-glucanase	25 BGU
Maltase	200 DP	L. acidophilus	250 million CFU
Glucoamylase	50 AGU		

*High Protease Formula three times daily between meals

Purpose: To help support immune function and assist in removing viruses, fungal forms, toxins, bacteria, and heavy metals
Each capsule should contain approximately:

Protease blend	150,000 HUT	Serratiopeptidase	25,000 units
Mucolase	8 mg	Nattokinase blend	400 FU
Catalase	50 baker units		

Nattokinase Formula three times daily between meals

Purpose: To support cardiovascular health and decrease blood pressure by breaking down fibrin
Each serving should contain approximately:
Necessary ingredient:

Nattokinase NSK-SD	1,000 FU

Helpful ingredients:

Amylase blend	9,000 DU	Glucoamylase	25 AGU
Protease blend	20,000 HUT	Lipase blend	1,000 FCCFIP
Minerals	85 mg	Cellulase blend	400 CU

Optional: Anti-inflammatory Formula for excess pain or inflammation

Purpose: To address inflammation, speed recovery, and repair tissue; best if enteric coated

Each serving should contain approximately:

Protease blend	120,000 HUT	Amylase blend	7,000 DU
Papain	140,000 PU	Lipase blend	600 FCCFIP
Bromelain	1,200 GDU (11.25 million FCCPU)	Catalase	100 baker units

SLEEP
See INSOMNIA.

SPORTS INJURIES
Sports injuries most often affect the soft tissues associated with proper functioning of the joints and general movement, including muscles, tendons, ligaments, and cartilage. These injuries include sprains, strains, dislocation or partial dislocation (subluxation), torn ligaments or tendons, BONE FRACTURES, and repetitive stress injuries. The most common causes of sports injuries are failure to warm up or cool down properly before or after exercise, structural abnormalities (for example, abnormal joint structure), and weak connective tissues. Some injuries can become chronic, particularly repetitive stress injuries.

Sports injuries are a very common occurrence and many of them can be treated without major medical intervention, the exceptions being BONE FRACTURES and torn connective tissue. After a sports injury, a series of metabolic processes often known as inflammation take place. One of the major concerns when treating inflammation is capillary blood flow, so the RICE (rest, ice, compression, and elevation) treatment method is usually recommended.

As the smallest blood vessels in the body, capillaries are responsible for carrying oxygen and nutrients to the cells and removing waste. After an injury some of these capillaries may be damaged, making them incapable of carrying fluid to and from the damaged tissue. This leads to fibrin build up and blockage "walling off" the damaged area. The result is pain, swelling, redness, heat, and loss of function.

To repair the capillaries, some type of anti-inflammatory drug (aspirin, ibuprofen, etc.) is often recommended. As a result, the bruises, swelling, and pain subside. The desired effect is to reduce the amount of fibrin in the damaged capillary, improve circulation, and speed healing. However, this can be done very efficiently with protease (proteolytic enzymes) instead of the usual drugs. Once in the bloodstream, protease hydrolyzes (digests) the fibrin network and enhances blood flow. Additionally, these same proteases have been known to stimulate phagocytes (cells that ingest foreign particles and debris) and accelerate elimination of work by way of the lymphatic system.

ENZYME SUPPLEMENTATION SUGGESTIONS:

*High Potency Digestive Formula with every meal

Purpose: To radically enhance the digestion and assimilation of food while reducing the body's need to produce digestive enzymes; the higher potency formula will average about three times the potency of the average digestive formula; an average formula may be substituted if three times the regular dose is taken

Each serving should contain approximately:

Amylase blend	22,000 DU	Alpha-galactosidase	450 GALU
Protease blend	80,000 HUT	Phytase	50 PU
Lipase blend	3,000 FCCFIP	Pectinase	50 AJDU
Cellulase blend	2,000 CU	Xylanase	500 XU
Invertase	80 IAU	Hemicellulase	30 HCU
Lactase	900 LacU	Beta-glucanase	25 BGU
Maltase	200 DP	L. acidophilus	250 million CFU
Glucoamylase	50 AGU		

*Anti-inflammatory Formula anytime there is pain or inflammation until healed

Purpose: To address inflammation, speed recovery, and repair tissue; best if enteric coated

Each serving should contain approximately:

Protease blend	120,000 HUT	Amylase blend	7,000 DU
Papain	140,000 PU	Lipase blend	600 FCCFIP
Bromelain	1,200 GDU (11.25 million FCCPU)	Catalase	100 baker units

*Serratiopeptidase Formula three to four times daily until healed

Purpose: To break down protein and reduce inflammation. Also supports cardiovascular health and enhances other proteases.

Each serving should contain approximately:

Serratiopeptidase	80,000 SU
Protease blend	70,000 HUT
Mineral blend	50 mg

Supporting enzymes:

Bromelain	Papain

For chronic conditions:

pH Balancing Formula before bed

Purpose: To help the body achieve an optimal pH
  Each serving should contain approximately:

Amylase blend	25,000 DU	Lipase blend	175 FCCFIP
Cellulase blend	6,000 CU	Pectinase/Phytase	200 PU
Mineral blend	Potassium bicarbonate, sodium bicarbonate, magnesium citrate	Herbal blend	Hydrilla, marshmallow, papaya
Protease blend	1,000 HUT		

The formula should not exceed 8.0 on the pH scale and the capsule should be enteric coated.

Optional: High Protease Enzyme Formula three to four times daily

Purpose: To help support immune function and assist in removing viruses, fungal forms, toxins, bacteria, and heavy metals
  Each capsule should contain approximately:

Protease blend	150,000 HUT	Serratiopeptidase	25,000 units
Mucolase	8 mg	Nattokinase blend	400 FU
Catalase	50 baker units		

STRAINS

See SPORTS INJURIES.

STRESS

Stress is a medical term for an imbalance in the body's systems caused by a wide range of external stimuli, both physiological and psychological. The body's physiological response to stress is sometimes called the general adaptation syndrome, which describes three stages of response: alarm, resistance, and exhaustion.

Stress creates an alarm in the body, and the system must retaliate by releasing certain hormones, such as cortisol, into the system to control the effects of the stress on the body. These hormonal releases create a cascade of responses, all of which are meant to calm the functioning of the systems and improve the body's ability to function in the stressful situation. Stress can have a major impact on the physical functioning of the human body by raising the levels of adrenalin and corticosterone. Long-term stress can be a contributing factor to heart disease, high blood pressure, and stroke.

If the body is responding to stress, then obviously other tasks within the system are either being stopped or slowed down. Therefore, symptoms such as indigestion, headache, gallbladder stress, and increases in heart rate and blood pressure may manifest. One way to control stress is to maintain a daily exercise routine, which is crucial to the health of every system in the body.

Recommendations include daily exercise, relaxation programs such as yoga or physical massage, and management and reduction of stressful situations. Enzymes can be used to improve digestion and circulation, support the immune system, and balance the pH levels in the body.

ENZYME SUPPLEMENTATION SUGGESTIONS:

*High Potency Digestive Formula with every meal

Purpose: To radically enhance the digestion and assimilation of food while reducing the body's need to produce digestive enzymes; the higher potency formula will average about three times the potency of the average digestive formula; an average formula may be substituted if three times the regular dose is taken

Each serving should contain approximately:

Amylase blend	22,000 DU	Alpha-galactosidase	450 GALU
Protease blend	80,000 HUT	Phytase	50 PU
Lipase blend	3,000 FCCFIP	Pectinase	50 AJDU
Cellulase blend	2,000 CU	Xylanase	500 XU
Invertase	80 IAU	Hemicellulase	30 HCU
Lactase	900 LacU	Beta-glucanase	25 BGU
Maltase	200 DP	L. acidophilus	250 million CFU
Glucoamylase	50 AGU		

*High Protease Formula before bed

Purpose: To help support immune function and assist in removing viruses, fungal forms, toxins, bacteria, and heavy metals

Each capsule should contain approximately:

Protease blend	150,000 HUT	Serratiopeptidase	25,000 units
Mucolase	8 mg	Nattokinase blend	400 FU
Catalase	50 baker units		

pH Balancing Formula before bed

Purpose: To help the body achieve an optimal pH
  Each serving should contain approximately:

Amylase blend	25,000 DU	Lipase blend	175 FCCFIP
Cellulase blend	6,000 CU	Pectinase/Phytase	200 PU
Mineral blend	Potassium bicarbonate, sodium bicarbonate, magnesium citrate	Herbal blend	Hydrilla, marshmallow, papaya
Protease blend	1,000 HUT		

The formula should not exceed 8.0 on the pH scale and the capsule should be enteric coated.

Antioxidant Supplement two times daily on an empty stomach

Purpose: To reduce oxidative stress
  Each serving should contain approximately:

SOD (superoxide dismutase)	75 mg	Catalase	250 baker units
Protease blend	50,000 HUT	Alpha Lopoic acid	100 mg
Glutathione	60 mg		

SUGAR INTOLERANCES

See DIABETES and HYPOGLYCEMIA.

SURGERY

Undergoing surgery can create a great deal of physical, emotional, and mental stress. Supporting the digestive and immune systems and improving circulation prior to and following surgical procedures can facilitate and expedite the body's healing. Due to the extensively varied attributes of surgical procedures and the medications that may be administered both before and after the surgery, it is best to consult with your physician regarding the use of enzymes and supplemental nutrients to be sure that they are not contraindicated in any way.

ENZYME SUPPLEMENTATION SUGGESTIONS:
One to two weeks prior to and until forty-eight hours before surgery; resume forty-eight hours after surgery:

*High Potency Digestive Formula with every meal

Purpose: To radically enhance the digestion and assimilation of food while reducing the body's need to produce digestive enzymes; the higher potency formula will average about three times the potency of the average digestive formula; an average formula may be substituted if three times the regular dose is taken

Each serving should contain approximately:

Amylase blend	22,000 DU	Alpha-galactosidase	450 GALU
Protease blend	80,000 HUT	Phytase	50 PU
Lipase blend	3,000 FCCFIP	Pectinase	50 AJDU
Cellulase blend	2,000 CU	Xylanase	500 XU
Invertase	80 IAU	Hemicellulase	30 HCU
Lactase	900 LacU	Beta-glucanase	25 BGU
Maltase	200 DP	L. acidophilus	250 million CFU
Glucoamylase	50 AGU		

*Nattokinase Formula three times daily

Purpose: To support cardiovascular health and decrease blood pressure by breaking down fibrin

Each serving should contain approximately:
Necessary ingredient:

Nattokinase NSK-SD	1,000 FU

Helpful ingredients:

Amylase blend	9,000 DU	Glucoamylase	25 AGU
Protease blend	20,000 HUT	Lipase blend	1,000 FCCFIP
Minerals	85 mg	Cellulase blend	400 CU

*Anti-inflammatory Formula three times daily

Purpose: To address inflammation, speed recovery, and repair tissue; best if enteric coated

Each serving should contain approximately:

Protease blend	120,000 HUT	Amylase blend	7,000 DU
Papain	140,000 PU	Lipase blend	600 FCCFIP
Bromelain	1,200 GDU (11.25 million FCCPU)	Catalase	100 baker units

SYSTEMIC LUPUS ERYTHEMATOSUS

See LUPUS.

THYROID IMBALANCE

See HYPOTHYROIDISM.

TINNITUS

Tinnitus, or "ringing ears," is a phenomenon of the nervous system connected to the ear, characterized by a perception of a ringing, beating, or roaring sound without an external source. The sound may be a quiet background noise or loud enough to drown out all other sounds. Common causes of tinnitus include presbycusis, prolonged exposure to loud environmental noise, and such pathological conditions as inflammation and infection of the ear, otosclerosis, Meniere's Syndrome, and labyrinthitis. Systemic disorders associated with tinnitus include hypertension and other cardiovascular diseases; neurological disorders, including head injury; and hyperthyroidism and hypothyroidism. Tinnitus may also be exaggerated by severe emotional anxiety or physical stress.

Some cases will resist all conventional modes of therapy. Since this problem is so widespread, the American Tinnitus Association (www.ata.org) was established to study and research the management of tinnitus.

Enzyme therapy can be used to support the health of the systems in the body that may be associated with the disorder, including the digestive and immune systems.

ENZYME SUPPLEMENTATION SUGGESTIONS:

*High Potency Digestive Formula with every meal

Purpose: To radically enhance the digestion and assimilation of food while reducing the body's need to produce digestive enzymes; the higher potency formula will average about three times the potency of the average digestive formula; an average formula may be substituted if three times the regular dose is taken

Each serving should contain approximately:

Amylase blend	22,000 DU	Alpha-galactosidase	450 GALU
Protease blend	80,000 HUT	Phytase	50 PU
Lipase blend	3,000 FCCFIP	Pectinase	50 AJDU
Cellulase blend	2,000 CU	Xylanase	500 XU
Invertase	80 IAU	Hemicellulase	30 HCU
Lactase	900 LacU	Beta-glucanase	25 BGU
Maltase	200 DP	*L. acidophilus*	250 million CFU
Glucoamylase	50 AGU		

*High Lipase Formula three times daily

Purpose: To improve fat digestion and metabolism, as well as the health of the cardio-vascular system
Each capsule should contain approximately:

Lipase blend	5,000 FCCFIP	Protease blend	20,000 HUT
Amylase blend	10,000 DU	Lactase	300 LacU

High Protease Formula three times daily

Purpose: To help support immune function and assist in removing viruses, fungal forms, toxins, bacteria, and heavy metals
Each capsule should contain approximately:

Protease blend	150,000 HUT	Serratiopeptidase	25,000 units
Mucolase	8 mg	Nattokinase blend	400 FU
Catalase	50 baker units		

TRIGLYCERIDES (ELEVATED)

Triglycerides are compounds consisting of three molecules of fatty acids bound with one molecule of glycerol. Triglycerides play an important role in metabolism as energy sources. They contain more than twice as much energy as carbohydrates or proteins. Elevated blood triglycerides are now considered as important as high cholesterol in the development of ischemic heart disease.

In the intestines, triglycerides are split into glycerol and fatty acids, and with the help of lipases and bile secretions, they move into the blood vessels. There they are rebuilt from their fragments and become constituents of lipoproteins, which deliver the fatty acids to and from fat cells, among other functions. Fat cells synthesize and store triglycerides.

There are two types of triglycerides: medium chain triglycerides (MCT) and long chain triglycerides (LCT). The body uses these two types of triglycerides very differently. Research has indicated that MCTs do not promote weight gain and burn energy rapidly, promoting both weight loss and the burning of LCTs. LCTs, on the other hand, are difficult for the body to metabolize, despite being the most abundant fats in nature. Therefore these compounds are usually stored in the fat deposits of the body.

The normal ranges for triglycerides in the blood are 60–160 for men and 35–135 for women. Elevated triglyceride levels have been associated with coronary artery disease.

Recommendations for lowering triglyceride levels include dietary changes to lower fat intake and regular exercise. Enzymes can be used to improve digestion, particularly the digestion of fats; improve the breakdown of fats in the body; and improve cardiovascular health.

ENZYME SUPPLEMENTATION SUGGESTIONS:

*High Potency Digestive Formula

Purpose: To radically enhance the digestion and assimilation of food while reducing the body's need to produce digestive enzymes; the higher potency formula will average about three times the potency of the average digestive formula; an average formula may be substituted if three times the regular dose is taken
    Each serving should contain approximately:

Amylase blend	22,000 DU	Alpha-galactosidase	450 GALU
Protease blend	80,000 HUT	Phytase	50 PU
Lipase blend	3,000 FCCFIP	Pectinase	50 AJDU
Cellulase blend	2,000 CU	Xylanase	500 XU
Invertase	80 IAU	Hemicellulase	30 HCU
Lactase	900 LacU	Beta-glucanase	25 BGU
Maltase	200 DP	L. acidophilus	250 million CFU
Glucoamylase	50 AGU		

*High Lipase Formula three times daily

Purpose: To improve fat digestion and metabolism, as well as the health of the cardiovascular system
    Each capsule should contain approximately:

Lipase blend	5,000 FCCFIP	Protease blend	20,000 HUT
Amylase blend	10,000 DU	Lactase	300 LacU

*Nattokinase Formula three times daily

Purpose: To support cardiovascular health and decrease blood pressure by breaking down fibrin
    Each serving should contain approximately:
    Necessary ingredient:

Nattokinase NSK-SD	1,000 FU

Helpful ingredients:

Amylase blend	9,000 DU	Glucoamylase	25 AGU
Protease blend	20,000 HUT	Lipase blend	1,000 FCCFIP
Minerals	85 mg	Cellulase blend	400 CU

ULCERS

See PEPTIC ULCERS or SKIN ULCERS.

VAGINITIS

See CANDIDIASIS.

VIRAL INFECTIONS

Viruses are one of the most frequent causes of infections. Because of their minute, microscopic sizes, these organisms can pass through even the tiniest cellular filters of the body. Once they enter the body, these opportunistic organisms make use of the existing cell host's enzymes and molecules to create more virus particles.

Symptoms of viral infection include fever, muscle aches, chills, and headaches. Examples of viral infections include the common COLD, INFLUENZA, tonsillitis, measles, certain BLADDER INFECTIONS, smallpox, encephalitis, croup, AIDS, cold sores (HERPES VIRUS), and mononucleosis.

Enzymes can be used to improve digestion and support nutrient absorption, to promote protease in the bloodstream that the immune system can use to break down the protein-based viruses, and balance the body's pH levels to promote overall health.

ENZYME SUPPLEMENTATION SUGGESTIONS:

*High Potency Digestive Formula with every meal

Purpose: To radically enhance the digestion and assimilation of food while reducing the body's need to produce digestive enzymes; the higher potency formula will average about three times the potency of the average digestive formula; an average formula may be substituted if three times the regular dose is taken

Each serving should contain approximately:

Amylase blend	22,000 DU	Alpha-galactosidase	450 GALU
Protease blend	80,000 HUT	Phytase	50 PU
Lipase blend	3,000 FCCFIP	Pectinase	50 AJDU
Cellulase blend	2,000 CU	Xylanase	500 XU
Invertase	80 IAU	Hemicellulase	30 HCU
Lactase	900 LacU	Beta-glucanase	25 BGU
Maltase	200 DP	L. acidophilus	250 million CFU
Glucoamylase	50 AGU		

*High Protease Formula three to four times daily

Purpose: To help support immune function and assist in removing viruses, fungal forms, toxins, bacteria, and heavy metals
Each capsule should contain approximately:

Protease blend	150,000 HUT	Serratiopeptidase	25,000 units
Mucolase	8 mg	Nattokinase blend	400 FU
Catalase	50 baker units		

Serratiopeptidase Formula

Purpose: To break down protein and reduce inflammation. Also supports cardiovascular health and enhances other proteases.
Each serving should contain approximately:

Serratiopeptidase	80,000 SU
Protease blend	70,000 HUT
Mineral blend	50 mg

Supporting enzymes:

Bromelain	Papain

Optional: pH Balancing Formula three times daily

Purpose: To help the body achieve an optimal pH
Each serving should contain approximately:

Amylase blend	25,000 DU	Lipase blend	175 FCCFIP
Cellulase blend	6,000 CU	Pectinase/Phytase	200 PU
Mineral blend	Potassium bicarbonate, sodium bicarbonate, magnesium citrate	Herbal blend	Hydrilla, marshmallow, papaya
Protease blend	1,000 HUT		

The formula should not exceed 8.0 on the pH scale and the capsule should be enteric coated.

WATER RETENTION

See EDEMA.

WEIGHT CONTROL

Weight control is a major concern for a large percentage of the American population. If you are overweight, it is wise to be concerned about your health and important to learn healthy and proper ways to lose weight. The health risks associated with being overweight include increased risks of Type 2 DIABETES, heart disease and stroke, osteoarthritis (ARTHRITIS), GALLBLADDER DISEASE, high blood pressure (HYPERTENSION), sleep apnea, GOUT, pulmonary problems, and GASTROESOPHAGEAL REFLUX DISEASE.

The most effective and long-lasting ways to lose body fat require time and effort, but the benefits are numerous. (See also EXERCISE, ATHLETIC PERFORMANCE, and ENERGY/ENDURANCE.) There are no miracle pills or easy methods. For some people, obesity is related to certain enzyme deficiencies, particularly lipase, the enzyme that breaks down fats.

Recommendations include eating a healthy, well-balanced diet; drinking lots of filtered water between meals; exercising regularly; and supporting the endocrine and immune systems. Enzymes can assist the proper metabolism of nutrients, particularly fats or lipids.

ENZYME SUPPLEMENTATION SUGGESTIONS:

*High Potency Digestive Formula with every meal

Purpose: To radically enhance the digestion and assimilation of food while reducing the body's need to produce digestive enzymes; the higher potency formula will average about three times the potency of the average digestive formula; an average formula may be substituted if three times the regular dose is taken

Each serving should contain approximately:

Amylase blend	22,000 DU	Alpha-galactosidase	450 GALU
Protease blend	80,000 HUT	Phytase	50 PU
Lipase blend	3,000 FCCFIP	Pectinase	50 AJDU
Cellulase blend	2,000 CU	Xylanase	500 XU
Invertase	80 IAU	Hemicellulase	30 HCU
Lactase	900 LacU	Beta-glucanase	25 BGU
Maltase	200 DP	*L. acidophilus*	250 million CFU
Glucoamylase	50 AGU		

*High Lipase Formula three times daily

Purpose: To improve fat digestion and metabolism, as well as the health of the cardio-vascular system
Each capsule should contain approximately:

Lipase blend	5,000 FCCFIP	Protease blend	20,000 HUT
Amylase blend	10,000 DU	Lactase	300 LacU

*pH Balancing Formula three times daily

Purpose: To help the body achieve an optimal pH
Each serving should contain approximately:

Amylase blend	25,000 DU	Lipase blend	175 FCCFIP
Cellulase blend	6,000 CU	Pectinase/Phytase	200 PU
Mineral blend	Potassium bicarbonate, sodium bicarbonate, magnesium citrate	Herbal blend	Hydrilla, marshmallow, papaya
Protease blend	1,000 HUT		

The formula should not exceed 8.0 on the pH scale and the capsule should be enteric coated.

High Protease Formula three times daily for one to two weeks

Purpose: To help support immune function and assist in removing viruses, fungal forms, toxins, bacteria, and heavy metals
Each capsule should contain approximately:

Protease blend	150,000 HUT	Serratiopeptidase	25,000 units
Mucolase	8 mg	Nattokinase blend	400 FU
Catalase	50 baker units		

YEAST INFECTION

See CANDIDIASIS.

APPENDIX A

DETERMINING ENZYME POTENCY

The potency of enzymes is not measured in the same way other nutritional supplements are measured. The determining factor of an enzyme product's potency is the effect it has on proteins, fats, and carbohydrates. In other words, the quantity of food that an enzyme can break down or digest determines its potency.

This method of measurement differs from what most people are accustomed to. For example, when comparing two vitamin C products, the average consumer will typically compare the price and number of milligrams per tablet of one vitamin C product with another. When it comes to enzymes, however, it is not quite as simple.

On the following page is a copy of the supplement facts box from the best-selling digestive enzyme product sold in health food stores, Digest Gold, manufactured by Enzymedica. Observe how the ingredients are measured.

In this example you can see that the name of the enzyme is listed in the left panel and measurement of activity is listed in the right panel followed by two to four letters. The word *Thera-blend*, which follows the name of four of the enzymes, is Enzymedica's way of indicating that more than one of that type of enzyme is used.

Nutritional Information	
Serving Size: 1 capsule	
Capsules Per Container: 90	
Amount Per Capsule:	
Amylase Thera-blend	23,000 DU
Protease Thera-blend	80,000 HUT
Maltase	200 DP
Glucoamylase	50 AG
Alpha-Galactosidase	450 GALU
Lipase Thera-blend	3,500 FCCFIP
Cellulase Thera-blend	3,000 CU
Lactase	900 ALU
Beta Glucanase	25 BGU
Xylanase	550 XU
Pectinase / Phytase	45 endo-PGU
Hemicellulase	30 HCU
Invertase	79 INVU
L. Acidophilus	250 million CFU
This product contains no fillers.	

What initially confuses most customers are the letters shown after the measurement of activity. On the Nutritional Information panel, amylase has 23,000 DU, while protease has 80,000 HUT. These letters are abbreviations for assays used to measure the "active units" of the enzyme. DU stands for dextrinizing units, while HUT is an abbreviation for hemoglobin units in a tyrosine base. The reason this is necessary is because enzymes are not measured by weight, and thus a measurement in milligrams (mg) or international units (IU) would not describe the true potency of the product.

Following are the three key factors to consider when determining the potency of an enzyme product.

1. Active units are the most commonly used measurement to determine potency, since they identify how active the enzyme is. An "active unit" is a measurement that describes how much of a given food an enzyme has the *potential* to break down. For example, one thousand active units of one type of lipase (the enzyme that digests fats) has the potential to release one

thousand bonds of essential fatty acids from olive oil per minute. When the lab technician tests the enzyme for its activity, however, she does so in a controlled environment in which the temperature and pH are closely regulated. To measure the activity of the lipase mentioned above, a lab technician will expose a measured amount of the enzyme to a fat (olive oil), in a pH of 7 at a temperature of 86 degrees to determine its active units. The measurement would tell you that the lipase has the ability to liberate one thousand bonds of fatty acids per minute, and it will be labeled 1,000 FCCFIP on the bottle. However, since the enzyme is measured using one type of fat in a very specific pH at a set temperature, the measurement is only an approximation of its potential to digest other types of fats in other pH levels or temperatures.

2. In the test mentioned above, one of the key factors in determining the potency of an enzyme is the pH in which the enzyme was tested. pH is simply a measurement of acidity and alkalinity. The higher the number, the more alkaline the substance; the lower the number, the more acidic the substance. pH ranges from 0 to 14, and 7 is neutral (the middle of the scale). The pH range of an enzyme is an important measure of potency, because it defines how long the enzyme will work in the body. All enzymes have an optimal pH and a pH range. When it comes to determining the potency of a product, it helps to know that one of the manufacturer's considerations was the pH in which the enzyme works best. This is important, since different portions of the body function at varying pH levels. The pH of the stomach averages between 2 and 3 (very acidic), while the small intestine is alkaline, with a pH of 8. The blood remains slightly alkaline at just over 7 on the pH scale. So, if an enzyme product contains a protease that has an optimal pH of 3, it will work well at digesting protein in the acid environment of the stomach, but may not work at all in the alkaline environment of the small intestine or the blood.

3. The third consideration is the number of enzymes used per category. Protease, lipase, amylase, and cellulase are actually categories of enzymes. Not all proteases can digest all proteins, nor can all lipases digest all fats. So the more proteases in a protease blend, the more protein it will be able to break down. A combination of enzymes within categories (multiple proteases, lipases, amylases, or cellulases) will digest or break down more protein, fat, carbohydrates, and fiber, respectively. This blending also increases the range of pH the enzymes work in and illustrates how one enzyme can break fewer bonds and be less potent than a multiple enzyme blend.

Obviously, there is a lot to the science of enzyme potency. Because of this, it may be difficult for the consumer to be certain of value and efficacy when purchasing enzyme products. Likewise, few companies have the expertise needed to produce properly formulated enzyme products that truly perform as intended. Therefore, I recommend purchasing enzymes from a company that specializes in manufacturing such products.

HOW MUCH ACTUAL PROTEIN, FAT, AND CARBOHYDRATES CAN ENZYMES DIGEST?

This is a complicated question, but note that every protein, carbohydrate, and fat is different:

- *20,000 HUT of protease* can break down 225 grams of dairy protein in one hour. Beef or soy would be different.
- *30,000 DU of amylase* can break down 100 grams of potato starch in one hour. The starch found in a carrot would be different.
- *1,000 FCCFIP of lipase* can break down 5 grams of vegetable oil in one minute. The fat found in beef or an avocado would be different.

A WORD ABOUT VALUE

When determining value you will no doubt try to compare enzyme supplement labels. Chances are the only useful information you will find will be the active units listed. Because the blending of enzymes is so critical to potency, you cannot assume that the higher the active units, the better the value. If you are comparing two products that cost the same and have the same number of capsules per bottle, note whether or not one contains multiple enzymes per category.

As an illustration, one product that contains multiple enzyme blends may contain 80,000 HUTs of protease, whereas a competing product with one enzyme type may list 100,000 HUTs. Despite the difference in active units, the 80,000 HUT product will be more potent since the blended product will work longer in the body and ultimately break more bonds than the other product. Which is a better value? In this example, the one with fewer active units but more enzymes would be a better value!

APPENDIX B

ENZYMES CAN SURVIVE STOMACH ACID

It is true that enzymes are affected by pH (the relative degree of acidity versus alkalinity in an environment). It is also true that on the extremes of the pH scale, whether acid or alkaline, enzymes can be denatured. However, many enzymes thrive in acidic environments.

Does the acid in the stomach, measured between 2 and 3 on the pH scale (very acidic), denature or destroy supplemental enzymes? The answer has to do with the source of the enzymes we are considering. Animal-sourced enzymes (trypsin, chymotrypsin, and pancreatin) come from the stomach, small intestine, and pancreas of animals, primarily cows and pigs. Since these enzymes are made from animal protein and become active in an alkaline pH, they are particularly sensitive to acid. This type of enzyme can be destroyed in stomach acid. But they can also be protected in order to survive the environment. All reputable manufacturers who sell this form of supplement enteric coat the enzymes. Enteric coating can be thought of as an armor that allows the enzyme to pass through the stomach unscathed and enter the small intestine, where it can begin to do its work in an environment perfectly suited for it. This is similar to the treatment of certain medications formulated to pass through the stomach without being damaged by the acidic environment and release once they reach the intestines.

One of the truly beneficial qualities of plant-based enzymes is that most of them are active in the acid pH found in the stomach. In other words, they are actually contributing to digestion while in this acidic environment. Yet what about plant enzymes that are active in a more alkaline pH? Do they become denatured in acid? No, they become *inactive* in acid.

You may recall from chapter one that enzymes will become either inactive or denatured when they are in an environment that is not conducive to them. The difference between these terms is that an *inactive* enzyme will become active again when the environment changes, whereas *denatured* enzymes have been destroyed and are now proteins with no energy or biological activity. It turns out that the vast majority of plant-based enzymes, especially those used in nutritional supplements, are not denatured in stomach acid; they are simply temporarily inactive until they reach an environment with a more suitable pH.

The National Enzyme Company (founded by Dr. Edward Howell) set out to prove once and for all that plant-based enzymes survive the acid stomach. They conducted an experiment, described on the website www.enzymeuniversity.com. I will summarize their study here.

Analyzing digestion of the same meal, researchers carried out four different tests: on the meal without the digestive enzyme blend under perfect digestive conditions, the meal with the digestive enzyme blend under perfect digestive conditions, the meal without the digestive enzyme blend with 70 percent reduced gastric and intestinal secretion, and the meal with the digestive enzymes under the impaired digestion model.

Samples collected at various times during the digestion process were analyzed for glucose and nitrogen content, demonstrating carbohydrate and protein digestion respectively. The enzymes improved the bioavailability of both proteins and carbohydrates in the lumen of the small intestine, not only under impaired digestive conditions, but also in healthy human digestion.

Glucose availability was increased fourfold in the "perfect" digestive system and by seven times in the impaired digestion model. Proteins were twice as bioavailable in the impaired digestive process. The activity of any digestive enzyme supplement in the small intestine "presupposes that the enzymes survive the acidity of the stomach."

While there are enzymes that are sensitive to acid and can be denatured in the acid part of the stomach (pyloric section), it is safe to say the vast majority are not.

IMMUNE SYSTEM 101

The immune system is a whole-body network of cells and organs which, when working as intended, defends the body against attacks from foreign invaders. These invaders include bacteria, viruses, parasites, and fungi. In general, the immune system protects the body using two types of immunity: innate, or non-specific, immunity and adaptive, or specific, immunity. Innate immunity consists of the physical barriers of our body, such as skin and mucous secretions. These barriers attempt to protect us from any possible intruder. For example, the secretions in the nose create a barrier to dust and all small particles we inhale, not just the pathogens that can make us ill. Adaptive immunity, on the other hand, is a direct response to a specific immune stimulus or antigen.

For adaptive immunity to work properly, the immune system must be able to distinguish between self and nonself cells in the body—those that belong and those that don't. Every cell in the body carries distinctive molecules that distinguish it as part of the body. This marker is its passport, if you will, telling the immune system it has the right to dwell within the body. Normally the body's defenses do not attack tissues that carry such a marker. Immune cells coexist peaceably with other cells in a state known as self-tolerance.

Foreign molecules, too, carry distinctive markers, characteristic shapes that protrude from their surfaces. One of the remarkable things about the immune system is that it can recognize many millions of distinctive nonself molecules and respond by producing antibodies that match and counteract *each* of the nonself molecules, or antigens.

An antigen is any substance capable of triggering an immune response. It can be a bacterium, a virus, or even a portion of one of these organisms. Tissues or cells from another individual's body also register as antigens with the immune system. Because transplanted tissues are rejected as foreign, people who have received organ transplants must take immunosuppressant drugs for the rest of their lives to prevent their immune systems from rejecting the organ as nonself.

How does the immune system attack and destroy foreign cells? The specific immune response is a complex system involving a variety of types of cells regulated by various organs and circulatory systems within the body. The organs of the immune system, known as the lymphoid organs, are stationed throughout the body and are connected with one another and with other organs of the body by a network of lymphatic vessels that are similar to blood vessels. Immune cells, or white blood cells, are conveyed through the lymphatic system in a clear fluid that bathes the body's tissues. Lymph nodes are small, bean-shaped structures that are laced throughout the body along the lymphatic routes. Found in the neck, under the arm, and in the groin (among other places), they contain specialized compartments where various immune cells congregate and interact with antigens that have been carried there by the lymphatic system.

The cells that are destined to become white blood cells begin as stem cells in the bone marrow. Some of them develop into phagocytes, large cells that devour or destroy harmful pathogens. One very important type of phagocyte is the macrophage. Known as "the big eater," macrophages are larger than other phagocytes and will engulf and digest just about any foreign agent and help clean up damaged tissues. They send biochemical messages to other cells in the immune system when they find and destroy antigens.

Another critical type of white blood cell is the lymphocyte. The two major classes of lymphocytes are B cells and T cells, critical elements of the immune system. The chief function of B cells is to secrete soluble substances known as antibodies, which are large protein molecules. Each B cell is programmed to make only one specific antibody. When a B cell encounters its triggering antigen, it begins a process that leads to the production of antibodies. Antibodies bind with antigens to identify them for removal.

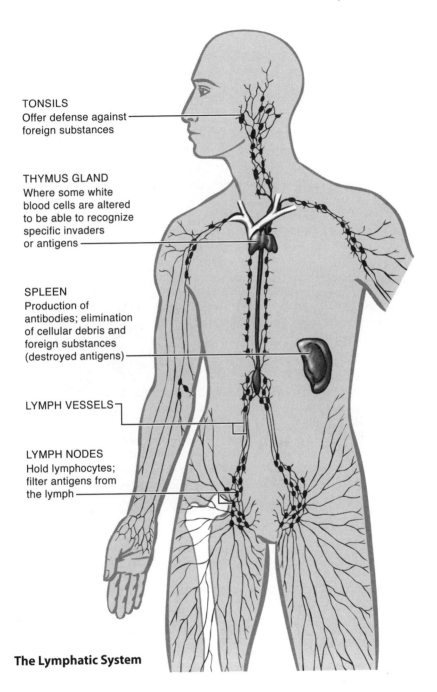

TONSILS
Offer defense against
foreign substances

THYMUS GLAND
Where some white
blood cells are altered
to be able to recognize
specific invaders
or antigens

SPLEEN
Production of
antibodies; elimination
of cellular debris and
foreign substances
(destroyed antigens)

LYMPH VESSELS

LYMPH NODES
Hold lymphocytes;
filter antigens from
the lymph

The Lymphatic System

T cells serve two major functions in the immune system. Some assist in regulating the workings of the immune system, while others directly contact infected cells and destroy them. The regulatory T cells contribute in multiple ways: Some activate other immune cells. Others act to turn off or suppress immune cells when the threat is over. A third type help rid the body of cells that have been infected by viruses, cancer, and other pathogens. They are also the cells responsible for the rejection of tissue and organ grafts.

Whenever T cells and B cells are activated, some are stored in the lymphatic system as "memory" cells, so the next time the system encounters that same antigen it is primed to destroy it quickly.

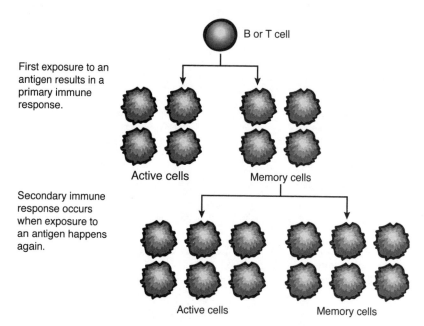

Some B and T cells are active and some are memory cells.

One way of understanding the interaction of cells in the immune system is that B cells travel through our bodies identifying pathogens and chemically marking them by producing antibodies. This alerts other cells of the immune system to remove the antigens. Several types of white blood cells are sent out looking for marked cells. Upon finding a marked cell, the white blood cell works to destroy it.

In addition to the primary system that controls our immune response, our bodies also have a complement system. The complement system consists of a series of enzymes that work with antibodies to destroy antigens. These metabolic enzymes circulate in the blood in an inactive form. The complement cascade is set off when the first complement molecule encounters an antibody bound to an antigen (tagged for removal). Each of the complement enzymes acts on the others to create a cylinder-like shape that punctures the antigen cell membrane and, by allowing fluids and molecules to flow in and out, dooms the target cell.

MOUNTING AN IMMUNE RESPONSE

Microbes attempting to get into the body must first get past the skin and mucous membranes, which not only pose a physical barrier but are also rich in scavenger cells and some types of antibodies. Next, they must elude a series of other nonspecific defenses, including patrolling scavenger cells, complement proteins, and various other enzymes that are part of the body's natural defenses. Infectious agents that get past the nonspecific barriers must then confront weapons produced by the body that have been specifically tailored to suit the intruder based on blueprints stored by memory cells after a previous exposure.

Long-term immunity can be stimulated not only by infection but also by vaccines made from infectious agents that have been inactivated or, more commonly, from minute portions of the offending microbe. For example, the flu vaccine is comprised of inactive flu virus. When presented to the immune system, the inactive virus acts as a Wanted poster, alerting the immune system to be on the watch for live flu virus when the body is exposed. Short-term immunity, on the other hand can be transferred passively from one individual to another via a serum containing antibodies. In this way, infants are protected by antibodies they receive from their mothers before birth and during breastfeeding.

In some situations, an immune response is mounted against some of the body's own cells when they become damaged or defective. For instance, when normal cells turn into cancer cells, their surfaces will change. These new or altered cells catch the attention of immune defenders, including T cells and white blood cells. According to one theory, patrolling cells of the immune system provide continuing bodywide surveillance, spying out and eliminating cells that undergo any malignant transformation. Tumors develop when this surveillance system breaks down or is overwhelmed by the sheer number of cells that have become malignant.

THE HISTORY OF ENZYME THERAPY

The history of enzyme therapy is fascinating. At times it is similar to a classic mystery—small clues over many years reveal the true identity and functionality of enzymes. In more modern times, enzymes have been the subject of studies on digestive issues, cancer, immune support, inflammatory issues, and many other debilitating diseases.

Though enzyme therapy has been around for centuries, those who used them did not know that enzymes were the reason a treatment worked. Two examples of such users are the South American Indians and the ancient Israelites. In South America, for example, papaya leaf was used to support digestion and promote healing. Papaya is the source of an enzyme known as papain; it is still widely used today for these same purposes. Moreover, the Bible (2 Kings 20:7) recommends the use of figs for boils to the Israelite nation. The fig contains an enzyme, ficin, which is still used today in some skin gels and dietary supplements.

In the Far East, there is an age-old tradition in which molds (fungus) called *koji* were used in the production of certain foods and flavoring additives based on the soy plant. Examples of this are *shoyu* (soy sauce) and miso, both of which are made from soybeans and originated in Japan. During the fermentation process, miso develops a complex and distinct flavor. Additionally, *natto*, produced from the fermentation of soy beans by means of a bacterium called *Bacillus subtillus*, has been eaten by the Japanese for hundreds of years. It has been credited with many medicinal properties and only recently have scientists given the enzyme found in natto a name: nattokinase. (See Amano Enzyme, Inc., "Natto—Traditional Japanese Fermented Soy Beans with Recently Discovered Health Benefits and Novel Industrial Applications," *Enzyme Wave* Volume 3, (June 2002): 2–4; "Prevent Heart Attack and Stroke with Potent Enzyme that Dissolves Deadly Blood Clots in Hours," Health Sciences Institute (March 2002); M. Maruyama, H. Sumi, "Effect of Natto Diet on Blood Pressure," Basic and Clinical Aspects of Japanese Traditional Food Natto II, 1–3, 1998; H. Sumi et al., "Enhancement of the fibrinolytic activity in plasma by oral administration of nattokinase," Acta Haematol 84(3) (1990): 139–43.)

In 1891 Dr. Jokichi Takamine filed patent applications for "Taka koji" from *Aspergillus oryzae* (a fungus rich with enzyme activity). This formed the basis for Dr. Takamine's fermentation process for the industrial production of a fungal amylase, the first of its kind. The method of fermentation suggested by Takamine is still used in the production of certain enzymes today. In 1894 Takamine moved his family to the United States and opened his own research laboratory in New York City. Takamine allowed the pharmaceutical company Parke, Davis & Company to produce his enzyme, takadiastase, on a commercial scale; it is still in use today as a digestive aid (Higasi, K., "Structural Chemistry," in Livermore, Arthur H., *Science in Japan*, (Washington, DC: The American Association for the Advancement of Science, 1965), 239–266).

In 1926, Dr. James B. Sumner was able to determine that enzymes are actually proteins. As a result of this, he successfully crystallized an enzyme, marking the beginning of commercial enzyme production and the use of enzymes as dietary supplements and food additives.

Elsewhere, enzyme therapy was heading down a slightly different path through investigations into the use of enzymes from animals. By 1930 enzyme therapy was moving in two major directions: the study of fungal enzymes, and the study of animal enzymes.

The following section is an attempt to credit the individuals who have been responsible for this research throughout the years. It is impossible to mention all of them, but here are some of the key players and their contributions.

THE FOUNDING FATHERS (AND MOTHERS)

DR. JOHN BEARD

John Beard was an embryologist living in Scotland in the early 1900s. His main research interest was the placenta. Beard observed that the cells that eventually become the placenta behave like cancer cells. He also noted that the placenta stops growing on day fifty-six of the human pregnancy, which interestingly is the same day the fetus's pancreas begins to function. He came to the conclusion that the fetus's pancreas secreted something that stopped the growth of the placenta and hypothesized that the same substance might stop the growth of malignant cancer.

Beard conducted experiments with juices extracted from young animal pancreases to test his theory. The juices were injected into cancer tumors and the tumors shrank in both animals and humans. Beard's work was published in the *Journal of the American Medical Association*. In 1911, Dr. Beard published a monograph entitled "The Enzyme Therapy of Cancer," summarizing his therapy and the supporting evidence (J. Beard, "The Action of Trypsin upon the Living Cells of Jensen's Mouse Tumor," *British Medical Journal* 4 (1906): 140–141). After Dr. Beard's death in 1923, the enzyme therapy was largely forgotten.

From time to time alternative therapists have "rediscovered" Dr. Beard's work and used pancreatic proteolytic enzymes as a treatment for cancer (Beard, *The Enzyme Treatment of Cancer* (London: Chatto and Windus, 1911). Today this same therapy is being researched by Dr. Nicholas Gonzalez, MD, who has published several studies on the effects of pancreatic enzymes on individuals diagnosed with cancer. You can read about his work at www.dr-gonzalez.com.

DR. MAX WOLF

Shortly after finishing medical school, Dr. Wolf was appointed professor of medicine at Fordham University in New York. There he became aware of the key role enzymes play in the vital process of life itself. He was one of the first to speculate about the therapeutic possibilities of enzymes.

He was able to convince Dr. Helen Benitez to join him from her post in the neurosurgical department at Columbia University. After conducting hundreds of tests, they concluded that enzymes were the missing factor for people who developed cancer. They also discovered that enzymes have an anti-inflammatory effect. Along with Dr. Karl Ransberger, they began to isolate many of the dozens of known enzymes that were responsible for anti-inflammatory activities.

After years of testing, they created an enzyme formula, Wobenzym (derived from a combination of their names, Wolf and Benitez). Wobenzym is composed of the animal-sourced enzymes pancreatin, trypsin, and chymotrypsin; the plant enzymes bromelain and papain; and the bioflavonoid rutin.

DR. FRANCIS POTTENGER

In 1932 Dr. Francis Pottenger began a study that ran for ten years, covering four generations of cats, more than nine hundred in all. In this study, Dr. Pottenger controlled the type of food the cats were fed. One group was fed only raw food and unpasteurized milk, while the others were fed a combination of cooked and processed foods. Dr. Pottenger then recorded his observations with exacting measurements and photographs.

The cats fed cooked and pasteurized milk developed common degenerative diseases such a diabetes and arthritis, while the group of cats fed *only raw food* prospered, living much longer than the cats from the other groups. Dr. Pottenger reported the underlying nutritional factor had to be a substance that was destroyed by the heat used in the cooking and pasteurization processes; the raw foods not exposed to this processing maintained this substance (enzymes), while the cooked and processed food did not. (See Francis Pottenger, Jr, "The Effect of Heat-Processed Foods and Metabolized Vitamin D Milk on the Dentofacial Structures of Experimental Animals," *American Journal of Orthodontics and Oral Surgery*, vol. 32, no. 8 (August 1946): 467–485; Pottenger, *Pottenger's Cats: A Study in Nutrition*, (La Mesa, CA: Price-Pottenger Foundation, Inc., 1995).

DR. EDWARD HOWELL

At the same time that Dr. Pottenger was overseeing the clinical study in California and Dr. Wolf was researching in New York, Dr. Edward Howell of Chicago was questioning the use of cooked and processed food for human consumption. He found that heating food to 118° F for more than fifteen minutes destroyed all of the enzymes that naturally occur in raw food. In 1940, Dr. Howell began to investigate whether or not chronic degenerative disease was a matter of a severe enzyme deficiency.

Dr. Howell wrote two books reporting his life's work: *Food Enzymes for Health and Longevity* and *Enzyme Nutrition*. Some of the most important and profound discoveries about enzymes and enzyme therapy are contained in the pages of these two books. The following are a few examples.

- Mammals have a pre-digestive stomach; he called it the "food enzyme stomach." In humans, it is the uppermost portion of the stomach. It is here that enzymes found in raw food pre-digest what has been consumed. When cooked food is eaten, enzymes are supplied from other organs to digest the cooked food. This produces a constant drain of enzymes from the immune system and other important organs.

- Any organ or gland will grow more cells and become larger if the demand placed on it exceeds its ability to function, much the same as a person's muscles will grow if they lift weights. Howell found that, in particular, human pancreases are two to three times heavier and larger in proportion to body weight compared to the pancreases of other mammals. He attributed this to consumption of an excessive amount of cooked foods, which place a large demand on the pancreas for digestive enzyme production. (William Donald Kelley, *Cancer: Curing the Incurable Without Surgery, Chemotherapy, or Radiation* (Bonita, CA: New Century Promotions, 2001); R. Weindruch R et al., "The retardation of aging in mice by dietary restriction: longevity, cancer, immunity and lifetime energy intake," *Journal of Nutrition* 116(4) (April 1986): 641–54.)

In the 1940s Dr. Howell founded the National Enzyme Company (NEC). The company today is one of the largest buyers of imported enzymes and manufactures finished goods for nutritional companies. While Drs. Beard and Wolf used animal-sourced enzymes produced from the pancreas of animals, Dr. Howell used certain species of fungus to grow highly concentrated plant-based enzymes.

ADDITIONAL IMPORTANT CONTRIBUTORS

GABRIEL COUSENS, MD, ND

Dr. Cousens runs the Tree of Life Rejuvenation Center in the United States and has written several books. My favorite is *Conscious Eating*, in which he talks about the importance of raw food, enzymes, enzyme therapy, and pH balance. In my opinion, this is one of the most thorough and balanced approaches to nutrition, health, and healing ever written. It is based on his experience and success in the clinic he founded and thus has real practical benefits.

ELLEN CUTLER, MD

Dr. Cutler, the "Enzyme Empress," as she is called by her patients, is the best-selling author of four books, an internationally recognized teacher, and an eminent public speaker. Dr. Cutler dedicates herself to further scientific research, teaching, writing, and ongoing consultation with clients with particularly complex conditions from around the world. Her latest book, *Enzymes, MicroMiracles*, is the culmination of her life's work.

During the past twenty-five years in clinical practice and subsequent to successfully healing her own life-threatening condition with enzymes, Dr. Cutler found that food sensitivities and improper digestion contribute to a surprisingly extensive number of ailments. These include obesity, skin problems, chronic fatigue syndrome, immune disorders, asthma, some forms of cancer, and of course digestive diseases such as colitis. Dr. Cutler's treatment approach incorporates her profound knowledge of both conventional and natural healing.

KAREN DEFELICE, MS

DeFelice has a master's degree in science and has written two books, *Enzymes for Autism and Other Neurological Conditions* and *Enzymes for Digestive Health and Nutritional Wealth*. She and her two sons deal with pervasive neurological and sensory integration dysfunctions, and have seen dramatic improvement in their conditions through the use of enzyme therapy. She has one of the most informative websites on enzymes (www.enzymestuff.com) and has never received any payment from any company for her endorsement. She speaks frequently on the topic of enzymes and autism and is an expert in this field.

HARVEY DIAMOND

Diamond's book *Fit for Life* is still the number one nutritional book ever sold, with 12 million copies printed in thirty-three languages. He is known as one of the greatest proponents of raw food and proper food combining. Diamond has shown through his personal life and his writings that one of the most effective ways to support optimal health and overcome disease is to eat raw food. In his latest book, *Living Without Pain*, he shows how enzymes play a crucial role in overcoming some of the most common diseases that cause debilitating pain.

DICQIE FULLER, PHD

Dr. Fuller's interest in holistic health began over twenty years ago when her daughter became ill and was given only a short time to live. She discovered her daughter's illness was a result of her inability to properly digest, utilize, and eliminate food.

With this new knowledge, her research turned to Dr. Edward Howell's work on plant enzymes. Her daughter began plant-based enzyme supplementation and experienced rapid and lasting results. After her daughter's recovery, Dr. Fuller began an alternative health clinic and a line of enzyme products used exclusively by health professionals, Transformation Enzyme Corporation.

Dr. Fuller was instrumental in my education and I have nothing but the greatest respect for her and the company she founded. Transformation continues to educate health care professionals on the benefits of enzymes and enzyme therapy. Her book, *The Healing Power of Enzymes*, describes common enzyme deficiencies, body typing, and practical dietary recommendations to support healing.

MAX GERSON, MD

In the 1930s and '40s, Dr. Max Gerson treated cancer and tuberculosis at his clinic in Germany. He was among the first to discover the importance of organically grown whole foods as he conducted research testing the reaction of all types of foods on the body's various systems. He found that raw ripe fruits, vegetables, and juices had the most healthful effects. Dr. Gerson believed that 80 percent of all disease could be eradicated by eliminating canned, frozen, and processed foods from the diet, foods completely devoid of enzymes. The Gerson Therapy uses intensive detoxification to eliminate wastes, regenerate the liver, reactivate the immune system, and restore the body's essential defenses, including the enzyme, mineral, and hormone systems.

RALPH E. HOLSWORTH, JR, DO, BSC

Dr. Holsworth has authored several publications related to the antioxidant properties of electrolyzed water and nattokinase, a fibrinolytic enzyme. He is member of the editorial board for the *Journal of Applied Clinical Thrombosis and Homeostasis* and of the Japan Nattokinase Research Association.

Dr. Holsworth has traveled to Germany and Japan in his pursuit of understanding enzymes in their clinical application. In Germany, Dr. Holsworth met with the late Dr. Karl Ransberger, one of the original researchers who determined the benefits of animal enzymes. In Japan, he met Dr. Hiroyuki Sumi, who discovered the nattokinase enzyme. Dr. Holsworth applies his knowledge and experience to support other doctors to understand the benefits of enzymes in a clinical setting.

WILLIAM KELLEY, DDS, MS

In 1963, William Kelley, a dentist, was diagnosed with pancreatic cancer. He rediscovered the connection between pancreatic enzymes and cancer remission (Dr. Beard's theory), and was able to cure his own cancer. He also subsequently treated hundreds of others with cancer. Kelley emphasized metabolic individuality, or metabolic typing. This theory holds that no single therapy, diet, or supplement is perfect for everyone, because each person's biochemistry is totally unique and different. Kelley identified enzymes as critically important and researched the influence of genetics on the autonomic nervous system. The goal of Kelley's therapy, which included a specific diet, nutritional supplements, and detoxification, was to achieve ideal metabolic balance that would enable the body to heal itself. (Kelley, *Cancer: Curing the Incurable*. Bonita, CA: New Century Promotions, 2006.)

ROY WALFORD, MD

Dr. Walford, a professor of pathology at UCLA, is at the forefront of the research regarding calorie restriction. Calorie restriction (CR) is the theory that by limiting calories to a minimum, the aging process can be slowed. The CR diet is one of the most extensively studied diets in the world. In one study, mice were divided into two groups; half were kept on a normal diet and half on a diet restricted in calories but adequate in everything else (R. Weindruch et al., "The retardation of aging in mice by dietary restriction: longevity, cancer, immunity and lifetime energy intake," *Journal of Nutrition* 116(4) (April 1986): 641–54.).

The maximum life span of the mice on the normal diet was 41 months, which would be equivalent to the maximum life span of humans of about 110 years. However, for the calorie-restricted mice, their maximum life span was pushed to 56 months, for a human equivalent of 150 years!

Similar studies on mice, rats, fish, and other species have been done in numerous university laboratories during the past fifty years, and they all agree: a CR diet increases the maximum life span characteristic of the species. It also increases the population's average life span, so the two together translate into longer and healthier life.

It is important to note that the reduction of calories is not the only criterion. The calories consumed must be "nutrient dense" healthy calories. (R.L. Walford, M. Crew, "How dietary restriction retards aging: an integrative hypothesis," *Growth, Development & Aging*, 53(4) (Winter 1989): 139–140; Walford, "The clinical promise of dietary restriction," *Geriatrics* 45(4) (April 1990): 81–3,

86–7.) Though I have never read or heard that Dr. Walford credits the lack of stress on the digestive system or the decreased amount of digestive enzymes required in a calorie restricted diet as the mechanism for success, he has said "CR increases DNA repair, definitely decreases oxidative damage, and probably increases the body's own antioxidant defense systems . . . Dr. Richard Weindruch and I postulated some years ago that the mechanism is related to an increase in metabolic efficiency"(Walford, "Calorie Restriction: Eat Less, Eat Better, Live Longer," *Life Extension Magazine*, February 1998). This reminds me of the role metabolic enzymes play in maintaining health within the body.

REFERENCES

Bailey, S.P. "Effects of protease supplementation on muscle soreness following downhill running." *Medicine and Science in Sports and Exercise* 31(5) (May 1999): Supplement S76.

Chichoke, Anthony J. "Enzymes Can Hasten Pain Relief," *Nutrition Science News*, 7 (Feb. 2001): 95.

Fuller, D. *The Healing Power of Enzymes*. New York: Forbes Custom Publishing, 2002.

Gardner, M.L. "Gastrointestinal Absorption of Intact Proteins." *Annual Review of Nutrition* 8 (1988): 329–350.

Klaschka, F. "Oral Enzymes: New Approach to Cancer Treatment." *Forum Medizin* (1996): 121.

Kleine, M., and H. Pabst. "The study of an oral enzyme therapy on an experimental erzeugre hamatome." *Forum of Practical and General Practitioners* 27 (1988): 42.

Kimber, I., et al. "Toxicology of protein allergenicity: prediction and characterization." *Toxicological Sciences*, (April 1999): 157–62.

Mamadou, Mahamane. *Oral Enzymes: Facts and Concepts*. Houston, TX: Transformation Enzyme Corporation, 1999.

BIOPERINE RESEARCH:

Eldershaw, T.P., et al. "Resiniferatoxin and Piperine: capsaicin-like stimulators of oxygen uptake in the perfused rat hindlimb." *Life Sciences* 55(5) (1994): 389–397.

Kawada, T., et al. "Some Pungent Principles of Spices Cause the Adrenal Medulla to Secrete Catecholamine in Anesthetized Rats." *Proceedings of the Society for Experimental Biology and Medicine* 188 (1988): 229–233.

Khajuria, A., U. Zutshi, and K.L. Bedi. "Permeability Characteristics of Piperine on Oral Absorption—An Active Alkaloid from Peppers and a Bioavailability Enhancer." *Indian J Exp Biol* 36(1) (Jan. 1998): 46–50.

Majeed, M., V. Badmaev, and R. Rajendran. "Use of piperine to increase the bioavailability of nutritional compounds," US Patent 5536506, 1996.

INDEX

www.Enzymedica.com

The role of Enzymedica is to offer the public the most effective enzyme products available. We utilize the expertise of doctors, researchers, and clinicians in formulating each of our products. And we have every batch third-party tested to ensure we always meet label claims. Enzymedica continues to research or fund research on the therapeutic effectiveness of enzymes.

Enzymedica's entire focus and purpose is enzymes. Our products contain the highest therapeutic activities available; no other company uses such high active units in a multiple enzyme line. And unlike most of our competitors, Enzymedica does not make vitamin supplements or herbal cleanses. All we manufacture is the highest quality, highest potency enzyme products available. In addition to the Enzymedica line, we manufacture and distribute Theramedix, a health professional version of Enzymedica products.

Enzymedica uses an exclusive Thera-blend process for its protease, lipase, amylase and cellulase. This means that each of these enzymes actually represents multiple strains. For example, there are actually four proteases in the Thera-blend protease. They are blended for their ability to break down numerous bonds of protein in varying pH levels. We do this at a considerable expense. From a label description Enzymedica also sacrifices active units to provide the best blend possible. A single protease, for example, could produce more active units per milligram than a multiple protease. However, the active pH would be narrow and the number of protein bonds it could break would be limited.

Enzymedica products are 100 percent vegan. Enzymedica uses no fillers in any of its enzyme formulations.